ER

Psychopharmacology and
Reaction Time

Psychopharmacology and Reaction Time

Edited by

Ian Hindmarch

Human Psychopharmacology Research Unit, University of Leeds, UK

Bernd Aufdembrinke

Schering Research Laboratories, Berlin/Bergkamen, FRG

and

Helmut Ott

Schering Research Laboratories, Berlin/Bergkamen, FRG

A Wiley Medical Publication

JOHN WILEY & SONS
Chichester · New York · Brisbane · Toronto · Singapore

Library of Congress Cataloging-in-Publication Data:

Psychopharmacology and reaction time / edited by Ian Hindmarch, Bernd
    Aufdembrinke, and Helmut Ott.
       p. cm. — (A Wiley medical publication)
    Includes index.
    ISBN 0 471 91818 0
      1. Psychopharmacology—Research—Methodology. 2. Human
information processing—Effect of drugs on. 3. Reaction time—
Effect of drugs on. 4. Psychotropic drugs—Physiological effect.
I. Hindmarch, I. (Ian), 1944– . II. Aufdembrinke, Bernd.
III. Ott, H. (Helmut) IV. Series.
    [DNLM: 1. Psychotropic Drugs—pharmacodynamics. 2. Reaction Time—
drug effects. QV 77 P97212]
RM315.P7498 1988
615′.78—dc19
DNLM/DLC
for Library of Congress   87-29469
                                                      CIP

British Library Cataloguing in Publication Data:

Psychopharmacology and reaction time.
    1. Neuropharmacology—Measurement
    I. Hindmarch, I. II. Aufdembrinke,
    Bernd   III. Ott, Helmut
    615′.78′0287   RM315

    ISBN 0 471 91818 0

Typeset by Mathematical Composition Setters Ltd, Salisbury, Wiltshire.
Printed and bound in Great Britain by Biddles Ltd, Guildford

Contents

List of Contributors

J. BERINGER *Institute of Psychology, Technical University, Darmstadt, FRG*

S. BÖRGENS *Institute of Psychology, RWTH, Aachen, FRG*

D. E. BROADBENT *Department of Experimental Psychology, University of Oxford, Oxford, UK*

P. CHERUY *Schering Research Laboratories, Berlin/Bergkamen, FRG*

G. DEBUS *Institute of Psychology, RWTH, Aachen, FRG*

L. J. FREWER *Human Psychopharmacology Research Unit, University of Leeds, Leeds, UK*

A. W. K. GAILLARD *Institute for Perception TNO, Soesterberg, The Netherlands*

R. GÖRTELMEYER *Clinical Research Department, E. Merck, Darmstadt, FRG*

I. HINDMARCH *Human Psychopharmacology Research Unit, University of Leeds, Leeds, UK*

R. IRMISCH *Clinical Research, Hoechst AG, Frankfurt, FRG*

M. JOBERT *Schering Research Laboratories, Berlin/Bergkamen, FRG*

G. KLEINDIENST – VANDERBEKE *Clinical Research, Hoechst AG, Frankfurt, FRG*

K. KRANDA *Schering Research Laboratories, Berlin/Bergkamen, FRG*

J. J. KULIKOWSKI *Visual Sciences Laboratory, University of Manchester Institute of Science and Technology, Manchester, UK*

D. LAMING *Department of Experimental Psychology, University of Cambridge, Cambridge, UK*

F. P. MCGLONE *Visual Science Laboratory, University of Manchester Institute of Science and Technology, Manchester, UK*

I. J. MURRAY *Visual Sciences Laboratory, University of Manchester Institute of Science and Technology, Manchester, UK*

J. F. O'HANLON *Institute for Drugs, Safety and Behaviour, State University of Limburg, Maastricht, The Netherlands*

H. OTT *Schering Research Laboratories, Berlin/Bergkamen, FRG*

N. R. A. PARRY *Visual Sciences Laboratory, University of Manchester Institute of Science and Technology, Manchester, UK*

P. M. A. RABBITT *Age and Cognitive Performance Research Centre, University of Manchester, Manchester, UK*

A. F. SANDERS *Institute of Psychology, RWTH, Aachen, FRG*

J. WANDMACHER *Institute of Psychology, Technical University, Darmstadt, FRG*

Foreword

In 1795 the astronomer Maskelyne, director of Greenwich observatory, announced the dismissal of his assistant, Kinnebrook, because the latter consistently required one-half to a full second longer to discover the passage of a star through the cross hair of the telescope than the director himself. It was not until many years later, when psychology slowly began to develop as a discipline, that it became clear that statements by two independent observers never coincide exactly, and that their 'reaction times to events' always differ by a certain amount, the so-called personal equation (Alechsieff, 1900).

In the age of mechanics of the sixteenth century, experimenters still used the so-called eye-to-ear method, i.e. by counting the strokes of a clock they were able to time in seconds the passing of a constellation through the cross hair of the telescope. Such methods were obviously not the most accurate and by the turn of the nineteenth century, in the age of electromechanics, it was possible to record reaction times accurately to a thousandth of a second using electromagnetic keys connected to a chronoscope after the method of Hipp. The invention of the kymograph with a soot-blackened drum made parallel continuous recordings of stimuli, reactions, and time markings possible.

Such technical methods were applied in experiments by Wundt, the first great German experimental psychologist. Moreover, and all the more remarkable, is the fact that great value was laid on the calibration of measurement systems *before* and *after* each investigation (Schulze, 1909).

The electronic age of programmable computers and the development of electroencephalography brought an enormous boost to experimental psychological methods in the 1970s and 1980s, particularly to the exact recording of reaction times to acoustic, visual, and verbal stimuli. These methods were backed up by modern theories of signal processing in neural networks, which dealt with filter properties in time and space and cybernetic models (cf. Bösel, 1981).

On 12–13 September 1985 a workshop took place in Aachen, West Germany, to discuss the theory, methodology and use of reaction time in psychopharmacology. Under the patronage of Professor A. Sanders, the contributions were collected in the following small volume.

ix

In 1979 the study group for applied technical methods (AAM), the initiator of the workshop, was integrated in the 'Collegium Internationale Psychiatriae Scalarum (CIPS)', which has published the three editions of the *International Scales for Psychiatry* (CIPS, 1983) according to its original concern of standardization of newly developed documentation systems and questionnaires within psychopharmacology. Together with a number of pharmaceutical companies, university institutes, manufacturing companies and other interested parties, the AAM has concentrated on the scientific adaptation and standardization of applied technical methods in human pharmacology and clinical practice. The AAM aims to evaluate current devices and methods and then give recommendations on pharmacosensitivity for the construction and application of specific concept-related measuring devices.

The first central theme to be chosen by the AAM involved the psychophysical threshold determinations of critical flicker fusion frequency and flicker sensitivity. The critical CIPS report, 'Flicker Techniques in Psychopharmacology' (Ott and Kranda, 1982), although published in English, has not found the expected wide audience, nor have the recommendations for a standardized, reliable, and validated measuring device for critical flicker fusion frequency been put into practice in the technical or commercial sense.

This deficiency points to the general difficulties that can arise and persist (for decades) when developing methods for this small sector of interdisciplinary collaboration between neurology, neurophysiology, psychophysiology, psychopharmacology, information theory, cybernetics, biometrics, engineering, and other disciplines. Antiquated concepts and technically obsolete devices are still handed down in applied psychopharmacology and the results are published irrespective of the latest findings from basic research.

In spite of, or perhaps even because of, the discouraging perspectives, the AAM feels pressed to carry on investigating and evaluating concepts of psychopharmacology and pharmacopsychology and to continue its endeavours for a meaningful applicability. The members of CIPS and AAM are always open to criticism and welcome all constructive comments.

The notion of a psychologically defined measurement of reaction time can, as apparent from the above-mentioned historical example of a star's passage, be applied as a ubiquitous concept for a number of stimulus response paradigms. These can be simple, like the simple response to auditory and visual stimuli, or complex, like multiple choice tasks. The simultaneous recording of different stimuli and reactions, e.g. visual stimuli, evoked potentials, the pressing of a button by hand or foot, as found in driving simulator models or in paradigms of visual evoked potentials, are signs of the latest developments based on the concept of polygraphic or multilevel measurements. They furnish information about the simultaneity of physiological and psychological processes and their chronological succession, and can be interpreted with modern theoretical models, such as the additive factors model of Sternberg.

This volume deals with such perspectives and documents methods and results from the field of psychopharmacology.

The editors would like to thank all authors and coauthors for their contributions. A special word of thanks goes to Prof. Dr. A. Sanders and Dr. K. Kranda for their active collaboration in this book. We are also grateful to the members of CIPS and affiliated companies for their valuable support.

References

Alechsieff N (1900) Reaktionszeiten bei Durchgangsbeobachtungen. In: Wundt W. (ed.) *Philosoph. Studien*, Bd. 16. Leipzig: Engelmann.

Bösel R (1981) *Physiologische Psychologie.* Berlin: Walter de Gruyter.

CIPS (ed.) (1986) *Internationale Skala für Psychiatrie.* Weinheim: Beltz Test.

Ott H and Kranda K (eds.) Flicker Techniques in Psychopharmacology. CIPS Report. Weinheim: Beltz.

Schulze R (1909) *Aus der Werkstatt der experimentellen Psychologie und Pädagogik.* Leipzig: Voigtländer's Verlag.

Preface

This book covers a broad range of topics. The 14 chapters deal with information processing—or to be more accurate, the speed and quality of information processing—and drug effects. But not every chapter examines both aspects. Indeed, the reader looking for quick and ready answers, perhaps even for cookbook recipes on how to analyse his own human pharmacological investigations of information processing, is likely to be disappointed. In contrast, those who, like the Editors, have had to find the hard way from the relatively theory-free application of simple psychomotor reaction time measurements to the construct-oriented application of the numerous possible measures of information processing, will find many ideas how to translate their research aims into reliable experimental designs. It should now be clear that we are not dealing just with speed, but also with accuracy, and a third measure, the speed–accuracy trade-off function, which combines both aspects (see Chapter 7). A further quality measure that is applied in road traffic research is the standard deviation of a vehicle's lateral position (see Chapter 14). Finally, evoked potentials represent a near-localization method of measuring information processing (see Chapters 11, 12 and 13).

We have placed the chapter by Kleindienst-Vanderbeke and Irmisch at the beginning of the book because it illustrates the classic use of reaction time in the research laboratories of the pharmaceutical industry. This approach is characterized by the routine application of a 'minimal psychological test battery' in the early stages of development of many psychotropic substances. Both simple psychomotor reaction times and choice reaction times are measured. The authors use multivariate methods of analysis (discriminant analysis, canonical discriminant analysis, factor analysis) in order to shed light upon the structures of their test battery and hence the starting points for the pharmacological effects on task performance.

The 'minimal psychological test battery' can be modified in different ways. In his chapter, Gaillard (Chapter 2) emphasizes the importance of criteria for the selection of test methods in drug studies and describes several alternatives to the use of traditional test batteries. These methods vary characteristics such as 'task', 'task variables' (e.g. signal quality) and 'levels' (e.g. intact vs.

degraded) which are assumed to have an influence on certain stages in the chain of information processing between stimulus and response.

Thus, in contrast to the analytical approach of Kleindienst-Vanderbeke and Irmisch, some authors can determine experimentally at which point drugs interfere with the operation of information processing. The additive factor method of Sternberg offers such a frame of reference. Interactive effects of the experimental variables, e.g. drug and task characteristics, indicate the influence of the same process, while additive effects suggest the influence of different processes. The pioneering work of Frowein is mentioned several times in this volume: Frowein was able to show that barbiturates influence the signal quality of a stimulus, whereas amphetamines act on the mediation of the response.

Not only the choice of suitable tasks but also the careful selection of the experimental design are important when planning pharmacopsychological studies. Ultimately, it is not the measurement itself which allows interpretation of the drug effect but the experimental variables which determine the occurrence and extent of the effects. The measurement of reaction times *per se* is of no value, it permits, contrary to popular opinion, no statement about general reaction performance. It is instead the operationalization of the time axis between stimulus and response in different possible constructs, which in turn determines the experimental design.

Debus and Börgens (Chapter 3) make a distinction between two types of experimental approach which they label 'state oriented' and 'performance oriented'. State-oriented approaches investigate the current individual *state* using physiological methods, subjective ratings from questionnaires, and occasionally behavioural measures. Performance-oriented trials deal with *changes of information processing*. Both approaches attempt to locate the starting point of drug effects via theoretical constructs. Because it deals with numerous different methods of measurement, experimental situations and subjects, the state-oriented approach appears to have greater external validity. In contrast, the performance-oriented approach, because of its stringent set-up, has greater internal validity. The authors are of the opinion that the bringing together of these two approaches, or at least their complementary use, would have the advantage of increasing internal and external validity of drug studies.

There are four chapters which in different ways make use of the additive factor method. The first two by Beringer and coworkers (Chapters 4 and 5) attempt to arrive at a greater insight into the interaction of information processing and chronological age. The authors do not necessarily interpret an interaction between task complexity and age as a *specific* effect of ageing. If the ageing effect—expressed as the reaction time of elderly subjects—is proportional to the task complexity—expressed as the reaction time of young subjects—then this could be due to a general slowing factor in the information processing system (complexity hypothesis). The reaction time of elderly persons is regarded here as a linear function of the reaction time of younger subjects with a slope greater than 1 (linear age function). The quality with which the reaction time of elderly persons can be predicted from that of young subjects is regarded as proof (for or against the validity) of the complexity hypothesis. An overview of the literature shows that the complexity hypothesis satisfactorily explains ageing deficits in which physical stimulus uncertainty or selectable processing strategies play no role.

In the second chapter Beringer and coworkers describe a visual search task in which they vary the automaticity of search and response decision processes. In the author's opinion the results of this experiment prove that the complexity hypothesis can basically be applied also to automatic processes. However, various ageing functions result for each separate target, which show additional selection mechanisms, such as physical uncertainty of the stimulus or semantic categories, are operating.

Laming (Chapter 6) also makes reference to the additive factor method, to which he applies a different psychological interpretation. His analysis is directed at empirically discernible fluctuations of choice reactions dependent on previous events such as stimuli, errors, and latencies. In contrast to the additive factor model, Laming interprets the still unknown mechanisms underlying these fluctuations, not as canonical components in the sense of successive stages en route from the stimulus to externally observable reactions, but as boundary conditions for the solution of a partial differential equation. He can thus depict effects as 'trial-to-trial' feedback following an error with just slight assumptions about the underlying process. The sequential effects of this experimental variable permit simple quantitative models, which for this very reason could provide useful candidates for the effects of drugs on reaction time. In this chapter Laming refers to his own—admittedly still unrepresentative—two-choice reaction experiments. The very high number of repeated measurements necessary for group trials is, however, a disadvantage.

Rabbitt (Chapter 7) reviews seven experiments which test the limits to which the use of simple measures of information processing rate can be taken for the assessment of the effects of age, alcohol, and individual differences in intelligence on performance of tests of reaction time and recognition memory efficiency. The index of the information processing rate—response speed or accuracy—is affected to a variable extent in an experiment depending both on the volunteer's interpretation of experimental instructions and the degrees of freedom that the experiment allows. Response speed and accuracy can be traded off against each other, depending on an individual's strategy. In Rabbitt's opinion true changes in the rate of information processing can only be determined in the relationship between speed and accuracy, the so-called speed–accuracy trade-off function (SATOF). He criticizes the view of the human information processing system as a completely passive mechanism in which a linear sequence of discrete non-overlapping and successive transactions are determined and proceed uninfluenced by other factors. In his opinion persons actively control information processing in continuous serial-choice reaction time tasks. The boundary conditions for this active control are determined by three parameters: the slope of the SATOF, which is directly related to the information processing rate: the reliability of error detection, without which no feedback for the selection of the lower speed limit would be possible; and the efficiency of the control of reaction speed. Taking memory experiments as an example, Rabbitt attempts to prove that reduced information processing speed is an important, but not the most important, factor in cognitive performance: 'There is more to being clever than being fast ... There is more to being old than just being slow.' This leads to the important theoretical, but also practical, conclusion that measurements of choice reaction time cannot be interpreted directly as indices for the efficiency of fundamental neuronal processes. A reduction of the mean choice reaction time under training conditions therefore does not mean that subjects learn to respond more quickly but that they learn to give more fast and fewer slow responses.

Broadbent (Chapter 8) suggests a short-lasting reaction time task with distractors, which measures two different types of selective attentiveness. Complex tasks that are geared to several neuronal tasks are not suitable for testing drug effects, because there is a danger of mutual compensation among the subsystems. For instance, noise improves the speed of reactions to a probable signal, but prolongs reaction times to improbable signals. A global measure would thus show hardly any change. Other aspects of performance refer to the distinction between the average speed for each task and the frequency of short periods of insufficiency. The latter are particularly evident in longer-lasting tasks. Broadbent suggests that drugs, but also trial conditions, be separated into two groups: those that act more on the average speed and those that influence more the variability of reactions and the occurrence of errors. It would, therefore, be desirable to have a task that could register a great number of such measures of attentiveness without necessarily lasting a long time. The task put forward by Broadbent is in two parts. In the first part the location of the reaction stimulus is determined, but not in the second. The difference in the two mean reaction times thus measures the relative advantage of a strategy of selective response over a strategy of scanning. There are correlations to external criteria such as personality measures and questionnaires on cognitive performance. Other feasible scores are the measure of compatibility effects, effects of distractors that are unrelated to possible responses, response repetition effects, effects of repetition of the location of the unknown signal, and right- or left-handedness.

Frewer and Hindmarch (Chapter 9) subdivide choice reaction time into lift-off time and movement time in order to investigate effects of time of day, age, and anxiety. They hypothesize that, compared with young persons, the lift-off time, which they consider the 'central' component in the reaction process, is more likely to increase in young anxious and normal elderly persons than movement time. Moreover, they expect a circadian course of reaction performance in the group of young persons, and deviations in the two other groups. No such circadian course could be confirmed in the normal group. In the two 'pathological' groups the reaction time was indeed longer than in the young normals, but this could be attributed to a prolongation of lift-off time only in the group of young anxious subjects. The authors at any rate consider it experimentally fruitful to separate overall reaction time into subcomponents.

So far the chapters have presented the reader exclusively with laboratory tasks. Sanders (Chapter 10) looks into the validity of these tasks for real life situations such as traffic safety, industrial safety, and household accidents and thus goes beyond the domain of pure laboratory research. He argues for an interactive process between laboratory tasks and 'field' or simulator tasks. In his opinion a validation of laboratory tasks in field processes would contribute to an increased predictability of the former, and would not only state more precisely under what conditions it occurs, but also under what conditions it is absent. The current standardized tests that refer to such practical aspects as job analysis, personnel selection and training either do not have an adequate theoretical basis or have too little empirical validation.

With regard to speed and accuracy, Sanders favours the first. Reaction times as independent measures are unproblematic as far as ceiling effects are concerned. They also require fewer repetitions as accuracy measures. Problems can arise, however, from the trade-off between speed and accuracy.

Kranda and coworkers (Chapter 11) are of the opinion that reaction times offer little information about the mechanisms of signal processing, since they cannot identify the neuronal processes involved. Nor can they differentiate central effects from peripheral effects, or cognitive from motivational influences. The authors therefore suggest the simultaneous recording of reaction times and evoked potentials to give an economical localization and identification of the different neuronal processes. They describe a methodology that can be applied to investigate not only brain functions, but also drug effects. The investigations reveal that the electric brain potentials to the forced choice detection of sine wave gratings of 6 c/deg can reflect, and in part separate, several different influences on the late components of an evoked response.

McGlone and coworkers (Chapter 12) used pairs of amoeboid shapes or vertical lines as stimulus material in a forced choice discrimination task. As early as 3–4 hours after benzodiazepine administration, while the plasma levels were still rising, they noticed a transient 30–40% reduction of the evoked potentials accompanied by a slightly longer-lasting prolongation of reaction times. Upon reaching the final plasma levels, these effects were already much reduced.

Similar observations were made by Parry and coworkers (Chapter 13). They report on the presentation of stimuli to investigate the processing of isoluminant chromatic and achromatic information and on the use of this method, together with measurements of reaction times, in drug studies. It once again becomes clear that one must use stimulus characteristics that allow a clear distinction between different operations of information processing. Taking a benzodiazepine as an example, they show that the processing of chromatic and achromatic stimuli is reduced by the substance in a similar manner and that this is not a selective process. Once again, the measurements of reaction times and evoked potentials are taken as two complementary measurements of information processing. The small number of subjects in the three studies shows that these methods are still at the beginning of their development; but they promise to deliver some exciting new insights.

In the last chapter, O'Hanlon describes an interaction, in Sander's sense between a field study and an analytical approach based on the sedative-related deviations in the lateral position during high-speed uninterrupted vehicle operation. This phenomenon is sufficiently well documented and reliable, yet it still awaits theoretical interpretation with regard to the underlying information processing operations. Three models are presented: the crossover model, modifications of the crossover model which consider potential discontinuities, and the Supervisory Driver Model. All three models attempt to explain the known effects of sedative drugs on variability of the lateral position during road tracking. Each of these models of information processing makes different assumptions about the processes involved, and of course they cannot all be right. The model that can best explain the observed phenomena is presumably the best representation of road tracking behaviour. Its variables can be investigated accurately in the laboratory driving simulator, and actual driving performance test. They could also contribute to a better understanding of drug effects if their psychophysiological importance could be identified.

At the close of this book the reader will be impressed by the many possible applications of reaction time and related measures of information processing in psychopharmacology. This diversity can be increased at will with the aid of computers. Yet it should also have become clear that all measurements are ultimately operationalizations of hypothetical constructs and that progress can only come from the further development of models. Psychopharmacologists are called upon to give more thought to models that guarantee the validity of their measurements. This is a fertile path for collaboration between academia and industry, which in our opinion has still to be pursued.

I. Hindmarch
B. Aufdembrinke
H. Ott

Psychopharmacology and Reaction Time
Edited by I. Hindmarch, B Aufdembrinke and H. Ott
© 1988 John Wiley & Sons Ltd.

1

Pharmacosensitivity of the Simple Reaction Time Test Compared with other Speed Loaded Psychomotoric Tasks

G. Kleindienst-Vanderbeke and R. Irmisch

Clinical Research, Hoechst A G, Frankfurt, FR6

Introduction

The aim of the present investigation was to determine the degree to which reaction tasks were able to differentiate between psychotropic agents. Data collected in a series of clinical pharmacology trials were reanalysed statistically in order to investigate how far the reaction tasks used were able to differentiate between psychotropic agents. These trials were carried out in healthy volunteers as part of the routine development of new drugs over a period of several years.

To obtain a greater insight into their pharmacosensitivity it was necessary to analyse the correlation structure of the different variables measured in the reaction tasks. Besides the simple reaction time test, the multiple choice reaction task and in one case the tapping task—as an additional speed loaded psychomotor task—were included in the investigations.

It was not the aim to detect underlying factors of the tasks performed under drug free conditions, which may reflect different abilities of the subjects, but to detect factors which are typically influenced by psychotropic agents.

Material and Methods

The psychomotoric tasks

Three speed loaded psychomotoric tasks were included in this investigation, a simple reaction time test (RT), a multiple choice reaction task (MCRT) and a tapping task.

The simple reaction test (RT)[*] measures the speed and accuracy of the reaction to a known visual stimulus (light signal). The subject has to react as rapidly as possible to 30 such stimuli displayed within four minutes at intervals distributed randomly between one and eight seconds. The performance is characterized by four variables:

(1)   mean reaction time (cs)
(2)   standard deviation (cs)

(i.e. the standard deviation calculated from the reaction times to the 30 stimuli)

(3)   total number of reactions
(4)   number of false reactions

In the multiple choice reaction task (MCRT)[*] the subject is confronted with 525 coloured dots on a screen. Each dot is presented for 0.8 second, one dot at a time. Each dot's colour and its place on the screen is randomized (total time to display the 525 stimuli is seven minutes). Subjects have to respond by pushing the correspondingly coloured button as quickly as possible. The performance is characterized by four variables:

(1)   total number of reactions
(2)   percentage of correct responses
(3)   percentage of delayed correct responses
(4)   percentage of false responses

The maximal speed of oscillating movements of one hand is measured in the tapping task. Within 30 seconds the subject is required to tap as often as possible with a metal pin on a contact plate. [†] The tapping speed is the average number of taps per second. In order to obtain reliable results this procedure has to be done twice, the scores are calculated as the average of both measurements.

Compounds

Studies with placebo and compounds from five different classes have been included in the analysis: tranquilizers of the benzodiazepine type, hypnotics, analgesics, alcohol (blood alcohol level 0.8%) and non-sedative antidepress-

---

[*] Supplied by Bruno Zak GmbH, D-8346 Simbach, FRG
[†] Supplied by Biodata, D-6374 Steinbach, FRG

ants. New compounds were classified in advance according to pharmacological findings and clinical reports, but independently from the results of the respective studies. The doses were based on pharmacological findings and other relevant information. The classification and dosage of standard compounds was done according to literature or our own experience. All drugs were administered as single doses.

Origin of data

The data were obtained from several clinical pharmacology studies performed ·under standardized conditions in accordance with the Declaration of Helsinki (1975, Tokyo revision) during the routine development of new drugs.

The data can be divided into two parts. Part A comprises four studies performed in 1976/77 under the same standardized conditions, Part B comprises two studies performed in 1983 and 1984 following different protocols. Part A was used for the main data analysis. The four studies were performed as crossover studies with placebo and compounds from five different classes. A baseline measurement before and three measurements after medication were available from each study, comprising 549 observations from a total of 31 subjects (see Table 1). The first measurement after medication

Table 1. Observations in Part A and Part B

| | Observations | | |
Class	Before administration	After administration	Total
Part A			
Placebo	8	8	0
(training)			
Placebo	53	155	208
Tranquilizers	16	45	61
Hypnotics	26	61	87
Analgesics	7	21	28
Alcohol (0.8 per mill)	23	56	79
Non-sedative antidepressants	20	58	78
Total	153	396	549
Part B			
Placebo	10	20	30
Tranquilizer I	10	18	28
Tranquilizer II	24	24	48
Total	44	62	106

took place between 0.5 and 2 h (time 1), the second between 2.5 and 3 h (time 2) and the third between 5 and 6 h (time 3) after administration, depending upon the study design.

The two studies in Part B used for the extended data analysis were different in design and included 106 observations (see Table 1). In the first study a tranquilizer was compared to placebo in two independent, parallel groups with 10 subjects each. There was one measurement before and two measurements (at 2.5 and 5 h) after medication. The design of the second study, a crossover study with 12 subjects, was more complex. It was an interaction study with an intravenous infusion of a tranquilizer and a drug of a different type as a second medication 75 min later. In contrast to the tranquilizer the second drug was administered double blind according to a crossover design. In this investigation only the baseline measurements before any medication and the measurements taken 10 min after administration of the tranquilizer were included; no placebo values were therefore available.

Subjects

A total of 63 healthy men participated in the studies. The 31 subjects from Part A were aged between 27 and 54 years (mean 39.4 years), the 32 subjects from Part B between 23 and 55 years (mean 32.4 years) (see Table 2). The subject group of the interaction study from Part B was homogeneous with respect to age (19–24 years).

In all studies, subjects had to abstain from alcohol, nicotine, caffeine 24 h before until 25 h after medication. Apart from the experimental medication they had to take no drugs for at least 24 h before until 25 h after administration of study medication.

Table 2. Age distribution of the subjects

Age (years)	Number of subjects		
	Part A	Part B	Total
21–30	2	13	15
31–40	18	12	30
41–50	8	5	13
51–60	3	2	5
Total	31	32	63
Mean age	39.4	32.3	–
SD	6.3	10.5	–

Statistical analysis

The data were reanalysed for a new purpose. The studies had, however, not been specially designed for the requirements of the new analysis. They were mostly crossover studies following different protocols. The sample sizes of the studies, the administered doses and the measuring times may not have been appropriate in some cases. The drugs may not have been representative of the drug classes; there were some missing values. Nevertheless, the data were interesting enough in our opinion to justify reanalysis before planning a new study, for example to decide which variable set will give only redundant information for a pharmacological question and which psychomotoric variables will add new information.

The main part of the analysis was based on the correlation structure between variables. Correlation matrices should usually be calculated from independent observations. In the present case, the observations were not independent, as repeated measurements were performed on the same subjects under different drug conditions and at different measuring times. Correlation coefficients give a complete description of the relationship between variables only if the variables follow a multivariate normal distribution. Some of the presented variables however, follow a markedly skewed distribution; data transformation procedures were not used. In spite of these difficulties we considered the correlation matrices to contain valuable information for experiences with reaction time tasks.

As mentioned before eight variables were measured in the two tasks, simple reaction time test and multiple choice reaction task. In order to avoid singular correlation matrices and linear dependencies between variables, only five variables were included in the analysis: 'mean reaction time', 'standard deviation' and 'number of false reactions' from the simple reaction time test, 'percentage of delayed correct reactions' and 'percentage of false reactions' from the multiple choice reaction task.

It should be understood that the statistical methods were used as descriptive tools and that we did not perform any statistical tests on the significance of treatment differences. These tests were performed earlier according to the special design for each study.

The following methods were applied.

Discriminant analysis

A generalized squared distance from an observation to a class was calculated using the difference from the class means weighted by the within-class covariance matrix (and the logarithm of the determinant of that matrix as an error term). Each observation is placed in the class from which it has the smallest generalized squared distance.

Canonical variables
The first canonical variable is the linear combination of the variables that has the highest possible multiple correlation with the classes (coded as dummy variables). The second canonical variable is chosen according to the same maximum criterion but restricted to those linear combinations uncorrelated with the first canonical variable. In this way the canonical variables explain best the between-class variation.

Factor analysis
Maximum likelihood factor analysis and principal component analysis were employed. In both models the factor pattern was rotated to the varimax criterion.

Results

Pharmacosensitivity of reaction tasks: mean values

Pharmacosensitivity is understood as the ability of a measure to differentiate between drugs and placebo. In the main, the shortest reaction times to simple stimuli were observed in the placebo and non-sedative antidepressant classes (Table 3). After intake of alcohol leading to a blood alcohol level of 0.8% the mean reaction time was prolonged but the inter-individual variability was increased so that the minimum and maximum of all values occurred in this class.

A similar pattern was observed for the number of false reactions in the simple reaction time test (RT) (Table 4); on average most false reactions were observed after intake of 0.8% blood alcohol, and the least after non-sedative antidepressants. The inter-individual variability was again high for 0.8% blood alcohol and hypnotics.

Corresponding results were obtained for the variable 'standard deviation' in the simple reaction time test (RT) (Table 5).

Table 3. RT: mean reaction time, values after medication, dimension (cs)

Class	Time 1		Time 2		Time 3		Pooled values				
	Mean	SD	Mean	SD	Mean	SD	Mean	SD	Min	Max	N
Placebo	29.0	4.0	29.4	3.9	28.8	4.0	29.1	3.9	19.6	37.6	155
Tranquilizers	31.5	3.2	32.2	3.9	30.8	3.2	31.5	3.4	24.4	37.6	45
Hypnotics	30.4	4.4	32.2	5.2	30.9	4.7	31.0	4.7	21.3	40.5	61
Analgesics	31.5	2.2	31.9	3.2	32.2	2.9	31.9	2.7	26.0	37.1	21
Alchohol	33.6	5.4	34.4	4.0	33.4	3.6	33.9	4.4	17.7	40.9	56
Antidepressants	28.4	3.8	28.2	3.4	27.3	2.4	28.0	3.2	19.7	36.2	58

In the multiple choice reaction task (MCRT) no impairment of reaction performance was found for analgesics and non-sedative antidepressants (Table 6). The 'percentage of false reactions' (MCRT) was slightly higher for hypnotics and tranquilizers and markedly so for 0.8% blood alcohol.

The most pronounced increase in 'delayed correct reactions' (MCRT) was seen after hypnotics and tranquilizers (Table 7).

To summarize these results: all variables indicated a marked impairment of reaction performance after 0.8% blood alcohol and practically no impairment

Table 4. RT: number of false reactions, values after medication

	Time 1		Time 2		Time 3		Pooled values				
Class	Mean	SD	Mean	SD	Mean	SD	Mean	SD	Min	Max	N
Placebo	1.23	1.7	1.44	1.4	1.14	1.1	1.27	1.4	0	9	155
Tranquilizers	1.73	1.8	1.33	1.8	1.73	1.7	1.60	1.7	0	7	45
Hypnotics	1.57	2.4	2.67	2.6	2.00	2.0	2.00	2.3	0	9	61
Analgesics	1.00	1.8	1.43	2.2	0.71	0.8	1.05	1.6	0	5	21
Alcohol	2.85	2.2	2.12	2.1	2.72	2.6	2.66	2.4	0	8	56
Antidepressants	0.75	0.8	0.95	1.2	0.50	0.7	0.74	0.9	0	4	58

Table 5. RT: standard deviation, values after medication, dimension (cs)

	Time 1		Time 2		Time 3		Pooled values				
Class	Mean	SD	Mean	SD	Mean	SD	Mean	SD	Min	Max	N
Placebo	3.79	1.4	4.07	1.4	3.81	1.2	3.89	1.3	1.0	7.7	155
Tranquilizers	4.05	1.1	4.36	0.9	3.92	1.0	4.11	1.0	2.2	7.2	45
Hypnotics	4.65	1.7	4.20	1.1	4.38	1.3	4.44	1.4	1.7	8.1	61
Analgesics	3.71	0.7	4.29	0.7	4.30	1.2	4.10	0.9	2.5	5.5	21
Alcohol	4.71	1.6	4.49	0.9	4.35	0.8	4.54	1.1	2.4	9.1	56
Antidepressants	3.73	1.4	3.44	1.0	3.61	1.2	3.59	1.2	1.4	7.7	58

Table 6. MCRT: percentage of false reactions, values after medication

	Time 1		Time 2		Time 3		Pooled values				
Class	Mean	SD	Mean	SD	Mean	SD	Mean	SD	Min	Max	N
Placebo	2.36	2.0	2.23	1.8	2.40	2.2	2.33	2.0	0.0	10.8	155
Tranquilizers	4.00	4.5	3.82	4.8	3.19	2.9	3.67	4.1	0.4	16.6	45
Hypnotics	1.64	1.5	4.86	8.9	2.47	3.6	2.74	5.1	0.2	36.5	61
Analgesics	2.75	2.4	1.89	1.8	2.35	2.6	2.33	2.2	0.0	7.1	21
Alcohol	6.74	5.6	5.89	6.2	5.28	5.7	6.00	5.8	0.2	26.1	55
Antidepressants	2.25	1.3	1.79	1.0	2.28	1.4	2.10	1.2	0.5	6.4	58

after non-sedative antidepressants. For analgesics, tranquilizers and hypnotics, impairment was observed in some variables or at some measuring times.

Scatter plots of the variables 'number of false reactions' against 'mean reaction time' (Figure 1) and 'percentage of delayed correct reactions' (MCRT) against 'mean reaction time' (RT) for the class means at each measuring time (Figure 2) show that differences between measuring times are marked for the class hypnotics and less pronounced for the classes tranquilizers and alcohol. No relevant differences were observed for the other three classes.

Table 7. MCRT: percentage of delayed correct reactions, values after medication

Class	Time 1		Time 2		Time 3		Pooled values				
	Mean	SD	Mean	SD	Mean	SD	Mean	SD	Min	Max	N
Placebo	9.6	11.2	9.7	12.4	8.7	10.3	9.4	11.3	0.5	68.5	155
Tranquilisers	23.3	27.3	23.2	24.5	19.9	23.2	22.1	24.6	0.6	81.1	45
Hypnotics	8.0	5.7	28.4	18.1	21.5	18.4	18.1	16.8	0.8	77.9	61
Analgesics	5.7	5.6	5.1	5.8	4.6	4.3	5.1	5.0	0.4	14.5	21
Alcohol	20.0	18.1	13.2	10.3	11.7	13.9	15.2	14.9	0.4	69.1	55
Antidepressants	7.9	6.8	6.6	5.4	6.2	6.2	6.9	6.1	0.5	26.4	58

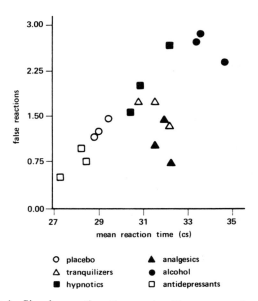

Figure 1. Simple reaction time task. Class means for each measurement (original variables).

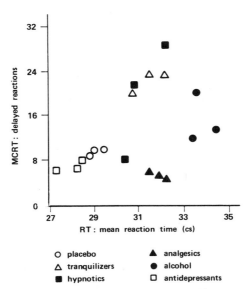

Figure 2. Reaction tasks: RT and MCRT. Class means
for each measurement (original variables).

Pharmacosensitivity of reaction tasks: discriminant analysis and reclassification

We have seen that the five chosen variables of the reaction tasks were affected by the drugs in different ways.

The drugs caused a general psychomotoric impairment or relative improvement as can be seen in all variables. Differences were seen in the onset, duration and intensity of the effects. However, the five reaction task variables were sometimes affected to a different degree.

The question arises whether these patterns are typical for the drugs and allow a classification of individual observations into the correct drug classes. Therefore, generalized distances from the class means were calculated, which took the covariance structure of the variables into account, and were used for discrimination. Observations were reclassified into the class with the nearest class mean; a high percentage of correct reclassifications indicates that the variables allow good discrimination between drug classes (Table 8). Better discrimination between classes of psychotropic agents is possible when taking different time profiles into account. The time profiles, however, may reflect different pharmacokinetic properties of the drugs in question rather than the common effects of drug classes. For example, the 100% correct reclassification

Table 8. Discriminat analysis using five variables of RT and MCRT. Each observation is placed in the class from which it has the smallest generalized squared distance. The table shows the number of correct reclassifications, expressed as the percentage of the true class frequencies

Class	Pooled values (all time points)	Values included			
		Time 1	Time 2	Time 3	Time profile[1]
Placebo	20.7	9.4	30.8	38.0	95.9
Tranquilisers	37.8	40.0	46.7	33.3	86.7
Hypnotics	4.9	39.1	26.7	34.8	100.0
Analgestics	85.7	85.7	100.0	100.0	100.0
Alcohol	43.6	45.0	52.9	38.9	93.3
Antidepressants	75.9	60.0	85.0	72.2	94.4

[1] 15 variables = five variables from three measuring times treated as separate variables

for the hypnotics when using the time profile instead of the respective times or even the pooled values, was probably due to the exceptional time course of the effect, and may therefore not be considered as typical for hypnotics in general.

Common factors underlying the variables of the reaction tasks

According to the results described above the compounds induced either general impairment of variable onset, duration and intensity or relative improvement. We were interested if the different variables broadly measure one general factor in reaction tasks or if different underlying performance factors are measured which can be affected by the drugs in different ways.

With canonical discrimination analysis it is possible to obtain new variables which best reflect any differences between the drug classes. These canonical variables are linear combinations of the original variables and may represent factors relevant for drug effects. With the present data we found two canonical variables of interest. Canonical variable 1 discriminates hypnotics from other drugs. Canonical variable 2 differentiates the drugs in a more general way. More or less all performance variables chosen are closely correlated with canonical variable 2 which therefore may represent a general impairment of psychomotor performance (Figure 3). The greatest difference in performance as measured by canonical variable 2 was seen between antidepressants and alcohol (Figure 4).

Methods of factor analysis (maximum likelihood analysis as well as principal compound analysis) did not show any essentially different results and are omitted here.

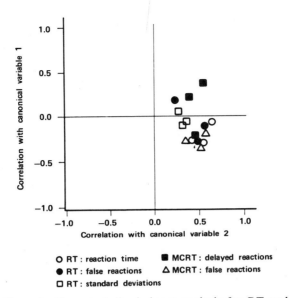

Figure 3. Canonical discriminant analysis for RT and MCRT. Data: pooled values after medication ($n = 395$). Observations: time profiles from three measuring times.

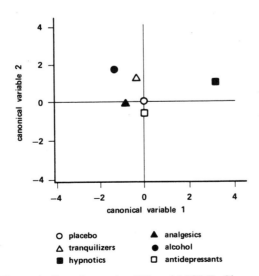

Figure 4. Reaction tasks: RT and MCRT. Class means on canonical variables (calculated from time profile).

Factor analysis of reaction and tapping tasks

The analysis of the first study of Part B (tranquilizer versus placebo) showed that it was again possible to extract one common factor which may be considered as general impairment of psychomotor performance. As the results were similar to those described for Part A they are not further reported here.

For the second study of Part B 24 observations before and 24 observations 10 min after intravenous infusion of a tranquilizer were available. For simple reaction time test (RT) only the variable 'mean reaction time' was measured, but another speed loaded psychomotor test, the tapping task, was performed in this study. Therefore four variables were analysed: 'mean reaction time' (RT), 'percentage of delayed correct reactions' and 'percentage of false reactions' (MCRT) and the 'tapping speed' i.e. the number of taps within a given time. Principal component analysis was applied to obtain two factors (Figure 5).

Factor 1 represents once more general psychomotor impairment (high loadings for 'mean reaction time' and 'delayed reactions'). 'Tapping speed' and 'false reactions' have rather low loadings on factor 1.

The rotated factor pattern (Figure 6) was obtained using differences from baseline as variables. 'Tapping speed' is clearly separate from the variables of the reaction tasks.

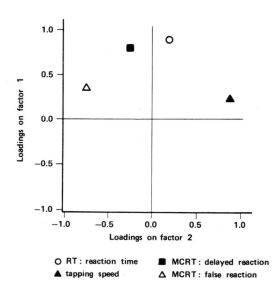

Figure 5. Factor pattern for RT, MCRT and tapping. Data: values 10 min after a benzodiazepine (i.v.: $n = 24$). Method: principal component analysis.

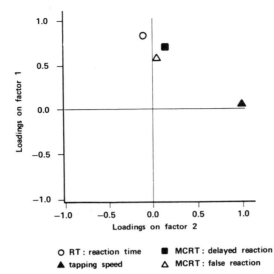

O RT : reaction time   ■ MCRT : delayed reaction
▲ tapping speed   △ MCRT : false reaction

Figure 6. Factor pattern for RT, MCRT and tapping.
Data: differences to baseline after a benzodiazepine
(i.v.: $n = 24$). Method: principal component analysis.

Discussion

To summarize, our results showed that it is possible to discriminate between
classes of psychotropic compounds using reaction tasks, especially using
variables of the simple and complex reaction task together. The best discrimination however was only possible when different time profiles were taken into
account. These time profiles however depend on the particular compounds and
not only on the drug classes.

We therefore tried to detect underlying factors which may be affected by
different drug classes in different ways and may be helpful for the classification
of psychotropic compounds. With the five variables of the simple reaction time
test (RT) and the multiple choice reaction task (MCRT), there was just one
factor found which represented general drug-related impairment of psychomotor performance. The pharmacologically induced changes clearly occurred within the same aspect of performance regardless of whether the visual
stimuli were simple or complex, with two exceptions:

1. A split between simple reaction time test and multiple choice reaction task
   was observed for analgesics: the 'mean reaction time' (RT) was increased,
   but the 'percentage of delayed correct reactions' (MCRT) was not
   increased. This may be the result of a technical problem as the reactions in
   the multiple choice reaction task may have been delayed but may still have
   occurred within the 0.8 sec allowed and did not therefore reach the

threshold used for classification as 'delayed correct reactions' (MCRT).

2. For tranquilizers a split between 'mean reaction time' (RT) and the 'standard deviation' (SD) was observed; the 'mean reaction time' was increased but this delay was broadly stable for the 30 stimuli, so that the standard deviation was not increased.

Nevertheless, it is worth stressing again, that a factor 'general impairment of psychomotor performance' can clearly be derived from a simple and complex reaction tasks.

The picture is quite different when 'tapping' is included in the factor analysis: the results for this speed-loaded variable differed considerably from those for the reactions to simple and complex stimuli. The drug-induced changes in the individual psychomotor speed contrast therefore with the change in performance required when instructed: 'react to external stimuli'.

This suggests that when performing reaction tasks under drug conditions the information processes 'decoding of the stimulus' and 'decision-making' on one side differentiate from the process of 'performing of the action' itself on the other.

As far as demonstration of pharmacological effects is concerned, it can therefore be concluded that it appears to be of less value to vary the complexity of the stimulus. More information might be gained by structuring the tasks according to the ' processing of stimuli' on the one hand, and on the other the 'performing of action' itself, which is one way of analysing the various compounds of evoked potentials, amongst other things.

Acknowledgement

We are very grateful to Drs W. Rupp, K. Taeuber and Mr W. Sittig for providing the raw data for Part A used in this analysis.

Psychopharmacology and Reaction Time
Edited by I. Hindmarch, B. Aufdembrinke and H. Ott

2

The Evaluation of Drug Effects in Laboratory Tasks

A. W. K. Gaillard

Institute for Perception TNO, Soesterberg, The Netherlands

Abstract

Studies in human psychopharmacology have specific problems of their own which are not normally encountered in human performance research. First, drug studies are more difficult to conduct, more costly and more time-consuming. The selection of the tasks and the choice of the design are most important. Since drug studies usually involve several conditions and sessions on different days, problems arise with regard to repeated measurements. A related issue is whether treatments are studied between or within subjects. In this chapter the various ways are discussed in which drugs can affect human performance. Drugs may have specific effects on certain psychological functions, and their influence may be direct or indirect via energetic mechanisms. Finally, some problems of interpretation are reviewed.

Introduction

It is surprising that there is no general agreement about the methodology to be used in human psychopharmacology. This paper discusses some methodological issues inherent in drug research with human subjects in laboratory tasks.

First of all, the type of task and the experimental designs used in the study of drug effects on human performance are very varied. In most drug studies, subjects carry out several tasks, and the experimental programme is repeated on different days. This can be problematic, since performance is liable to change over time due to practice or fatigue. Moreover, performance in one task can have a positive or negative effect on performance in other tasks, thus producing an asymmetric transfer (Poulton and Freeman, 1966).

15

Second, one of the most important aspects of a drug study is the choice of laboratory tasks, e.g., choice reaction time, vigilance, tracking, memory, selective attention. Drugs are often investigated in a test battery that aims to cover a large range of human abilities. Yet most tests that are used in batteries do not have a theoretical background, and this can hamper the interpretation of the results. A more specific approach is the one based upon the additive factor method (Sternberg, 1969); with this method only one task is used, and the drug effects on performance are evaluated as a function of two or more task variables. This approach yields more specific results, but it is only applicable to a limited number of psychological functions (Frowein, 1981).

Third, the training procedures and the instructions are as important as the choice of tasks or task variables. It is often forgotten that task procedures are probably more decisive in producing drug effects than the task itself. A significant drug effect in a memory task does not necessarily imply that the drug affects memory. Instead, the effect may be attributable to aspects of the task that are not directly related to memory processes, such as stimulus modality, task duration, or stimulus rate. The effect may also be so general that performance is affected in any task.

Fourth, it is recommended that measures of performance be complemented with questions on subjective feelings. Together with such physiological variables as heart rate, respiration, and EEG, subjective measures provide additional information about the way a drug affects performance. Since subjects are liable to vary in their responsiveness to drugs, inventories on personality or psychosomatic complaints should also be included.

Finally, the investigator should be familiar with the pharmacokinetics of the drug before determining the time frame in which tasks are to be carried out. The time course of drug action based on blood or urine samples, however, may not correspond to the time course based on performance, subjective feelings, or physiological measures. If there is any uncertainty about the behavioural pharmacokinetics, the same task should be repeated several times on the same day, say, one, three and five hours after treatment. In most studies measurements are collected over several sessions on the same day, so the effects of time since treatment, time on task, and time of day are usually confounded. In the following sections the problems relating to design, choice of tasks, and the determination of the nature of effects will be further outlined, and some suggestions towards a more general methodology will be presented.

Within-subject and Between-subject Designs

The effects of drugs are usually evaluated on the basis of performance in one or more tasks that are carried out one or more times on the same day. The investigator has to decide whether to adopt a within-subject (independent groups) or a between-subject (crossover) design. In the latter design, subjects receive all treatments, whereas in the former design there is a separate subject group for each treatment. The advantage of a crossover design is that each subject acts as his own control (drug vs. placebo). This is important because there are considerable individual differences not only in the performance level, but also in the responsiveness to the drug. Between-subject designs require large groups of subjects, which may raise practical problems. A disadvantage of the crossover design is that subjects receive several treatments, often at weekly intervals, and that performance on a particular day may be affected by performance and the drug effects of a previous session (Poulton and Freeman, 1966). Performance changes over sessions can be due to practice, to adaptation to the laboratory situation, and to a loss of motivation or interest.

Although it is generally accepted that performance can improve with repeated sessions of the same task, this factor is seldom taken into account. A related factor concerns the adaptation of the subject to the laboratory environment. For instance, it has been shown that heart rate decreases in both sessions on the same day and between days of testing. To overcome some of these problems a full day of practice is needed in the week before the first drug treatment; the programme on this practice day should be the same as on the actual treatment days.

A crossover design allows only a limited number of treatments. With three treatments and one placebo, the experiment already takes at least five weeks. At the end of the study subjects are liable to become bored and lose their motivation, and consequently they may find it hard to maintain efficient performance. Again, this is probably highly relevant with regard to drug effects.

Test Batteries and Task Variables

It is becoming more and more important to investigate the selective effects of drugs on mental functions. Simply finding an effect seems no longer satisfactory. The relevant question is which types of task are sensitive to a drug and, more importantly, which types are not affected by the drug. Knowledge of selective effects on tasks or task variables may shed some light on how a drug affects human performance and which mental functions are primarily affected by which drugs.

Test batteries cannot be used in this approach because most tasks have no theoretical background. It is unclear what most tasks are supposed to measure and whether one or several mental functions are involved. A good example is the Digit Symbol Substitution Test. In this paper-and-pencil test, symbols are translated into one of the digits 1–9 according to the instructions at the top of the test sheet. Depending on the interpretation of the investigator, the results may reflect a drug effect on the following mental functions: a) the perceptual encoding of symbols; b) the storage of the symbols or symbol-digit relations in working memory: c) the central process of translating symbols into digits: d) the selective attention to a position on the sheet while ignoring symbols in other positions; e) the control of eye movements back and forth across the sheet; f) the skill of writing down the digits; g) the subject's motivation, because the task is selfpaced and therefore vulnerable to lapses of attention. Thus, when a significant effect of a drug is found in this test, it is impossible to specify which mental function is affected.

The more general problem behind the choice of task is the lack of a taxonomy or criteria for selecting a particular task. In general, it has to be assumed that several mental functions are needed in any task, but some of them are more involved than others.

One way of solving the above problems is to apply the additive factor method (Sternberg, 1969; Sanders, 1980). With this approach, drug effects are studied as a function of task variables that are assumed to manipulate a particular stage in the chain of information processing between stimulus and response (see also Figure 1). Hence, Frowein (1981) found that a barbiturate had a selective effect on stimulus encoding since its effect (placebo vs. barbiturate) interacted with the effect of stimulus quality (intact vs. degraded stimuli): the degradation of the stimuli had a larger effect after administration of a barbiturate than of a placebo. A similar interaction was not found in connection with task variables associated with other stages. In contrast, an amphetamine appeared to affect stages related to response processing. Thus, both types of drug had selective effects, but on different functions.

As illustrated in Figure 2, there is an essential difference between the task battery approach and the factorial design required by the additive factor method: in the former, there are several tasks, but no task variables; whereas

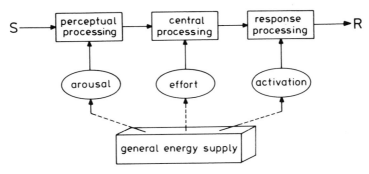

Figure 1. A schematic representation of a model in which structural processes are supplied by energetic mechanisms. Three processing stages mediate between stimulus (*S*) and response (*R*). Each stage has its own energy supply, which in turn is maintained by a general energy supply. This model is an elaboration of the models presented in Gaillard (1980) and Sanders (1983).

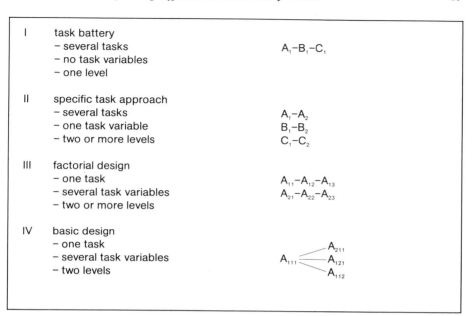

Figure 2. Four study designs used in psychopharmacology. A, B, C, refer to the tasks involved. The number of task variables is indicated by the number of indices; the index itself gives the level on the task variable. In a *task battery*, only one version is used of several tasks (A, B, C). In the *specific task approach* there are two levels (1, 2) for only one task variable for each of the tasks (A, B, C). In the *factorial design,* there are two levels on each of the two task variables (11, 21, 12, 22) within one task only. The *basic design* is a simplification of the factorial design, in the sense that the interactions are left out; for example, A_{222} is not included.

in the latter, there are several task variables within the same task. The advantage of using task variables rather than tasks is that the observed effects are specific and open to interpretation in terms of mental processes. Disadvantages of the factorial design are that it is rather time-consuming and is only applicable to mental processes that can be manipulated in a choice reaction task. There are various phenomena and mental functions that cannot be covered by a choice reaction time task, especially more complex aspects of performance. In contrast, test batteries are usually less time-consuming, are easy to administer, and can cover a wide range of mental functions. Figure 2 presents two additional approaches than can be used to study drug effects. The 'specific task approach' is an attempt to combine the relative advantages of the task battery and factorial approaches by having two levels on one task variable (e.g., signal quality), but in qualitatively different tasks. In this way, a wider range of tasks can be chosen, whereas the interaction between drug and task variable may still yield a specific effect.

The 'basic design' is a simplification of the factorial design. For each of the two or more task variables, the level of difficulty is manipulated, but tests concerning the interactions between task variables are not included. The basic design is an incomplete factorial design and is therefore time-saving. It also allows specific statements with respect to the localization of the action of the drug under investigation. As in the specific task approach, the starting point is that the stages of processing involved in the manipulations of the task variables are largely known from investigations in earlier studies with a complete factorial design.

The Nature of Effects

In human psychopharmacology, it is becoming clear that research should be directed to the question of how drugs affect mental information processing. An important step towards this goal is the search for selective effects on mental functions with the designs described in the previous section. The evaluation of ways in which a drug influences human performance raises the questions of how specific and direct the effects are.

The degree of specificity depends on the range of mental processes that are affected. As outlined in the previous section, a barbiturate appears to have a specific effect on perceptual encoding, whereas other stages, such as central processing and response processing, remain unaffected. Other drugs may have more general effects, i.e., performance is reduced irrespective of the task or task variable used. For example, a drug may slow down the overall processing speed and therefore have an adverse effect on all mental functions.

A common distinction in human performance research is that between structural processes and energetic mechanisms. Structural processes are operations that mediate between stimulus and response; they are thought to be dependent on the structure of the task and on the task instructions. Structural processes are always necessary for the execution of a task and, following the computer metaphor, are often referred to as 'computational'.

Energetic mechanisms, such as arousal, are not directly involved in information processing, but modulate the structural processes. These mechanisms have been conceptualized to explain the adverse effects of variables like sleep loss and time on task. The traditional idea is that an unspecific 'pool of energy' supports all mental functions. Nowadays most theories of energy or effort assume that there are independent energetic resources connected to different mental functions (see Hockey *et al.*, 1986).

Figure 1 presents a schematic representation of a multi-response view. Each stage in the chain of information processing has its own energy supply (Gaillard, 1980; Sanders, 1983). In addition, there is a general supply that feeds and maintains the specific supplies, depending on the type of task and the subject's strategy for allocating the general resource.

On the basis of Figure 1, various ways can be proposed in which drugs affect human performance:

1. Specific–direct. The drug has a direct effect on a particular mental function. The drug therefore has only an effect on specific tasks, or its effect varies as a function of some specific task variables.
2. Unspecific–direct. The drug has no specific effect on any particular mental function. The same effect is found irrespective of the type of task or task variable.
3. Specific–indirect. The drug has a specific effect on a particular energetic mechanism associated with a limited number of mental functions.
4. Unspecific–indirect. The drug affects the general energy supply and indirectly all specific energetic mechanisms and mental functions.

The way a drug affects performance varies with the dosage and the route of administration. For example, a barbiturate is liable to have specific effects at low dosages and general effects at higher dosages, even to the extent that subjects fall asleep.

So far, there are no generally agreed methods of distinguishing between direct effects on structural processes and indirect effects via energetic mechanisms. One way is to assume that effects are direct when they are invariably observed—even in normal, healthy, motivated subjects working under optimal conditions (Sanders, 1983). In contrast, effects may be regarded as indirect when they only emerge as an interaction with 'organismic' variables known to influence a subject's state and energetic mechanisms, such as time of day, time on task, task duration, or sleep deprivation. Thus, the effect of a barbiturate on perceptual encoding seems to be direct, because it has been found in subjects under optimal conditions (short task duration, etc.). The effect of an amphetamine appears to be most prominent in conditions where maintaining sufficient energy supplies is likely to be problematic, i.e., sleep deprivation and long-term performance.

Frowein *et al.*, (1981), for instance, found that an amphetamine had only clear effects in sleep-deprived subjects. One night of sleep deprivation impaired performance on choice reaction time in particular when the stimuli were presented at highly variable intervals. That the effect was fully compensated by amphetamine suggests that sleep deprivation and amphetamines both influence 'activation' (see Figure 1) which mechanism is assumed to supply energy for the response processing stage.

It has been claimed that the effects of ACTH analogues have a direct influence on learning and memory processes. It has been demonstrated, however, that the effect is only found at the end of a relatively long session (30 minutes), whereas no effect is observed when the same task is performed for a short period (5 minutes). This suggests that ACTH analogues compensate for inhibitory tendencies that build up over a long demanding session.

They therefore only affect performance indirectly via energetic mechanisms (Gaillard, 1981).

It is still relatively simple to draw the distinction between direct computational and indirect energetic efforts within the framework of additive factors logic. The issues become considerably more complicated in tests outside this framework. Thus, if a significant drug effect is found on, say, a memory test, this does not necessarily imply that the drug under investigation affects memory. The effect could be interpreted in the following ways:

1. Specific. The drug has a specific and direct effect on memory. This would imply that it would also show up in related memory tests.
2. General. The effect is found irrespective of the type of task or task variable used. Thus, it is also found in tasks that do not involve memory functions.
3. Energetic. An effect is only found in conditions where the energy supply is problematic and liable to be insufficient. The effect disappears when the test is carried out under optimal conditions.
4. Unknown factor. The effect is due to aspects of the task (presentation rate, stimulus or response modality, etc.) that are unrelated to the function which the task aims to evaluate. In this case, the effect will not show up in related memory tasks when the confounded aspects are different.
5. Random effect. The effect is due to a type I error, i.e., the null hypothesis is erroneously rejected. With a significance level of 0.05, one out of 20 significant effects can be ascribed to random fluctuations in the data.

In most instances, significant effects are regarded as specific, and alternative interpretations are not seriously considered. It is common practice to present empirical results in a too positive light. Editors as well as authors tend to be sceptical towards null results.

If the result of a study is negative, i.e., a particular drug fails to have a significant effect, there is a tendency to raise doubts about the competence of the investigator, the sensitivity of the task, the appropriateness of the design, or the number of subjects used. These all appear not to be relevant in studies with positive results. This tendency is even more prominent in human psychopharmacological studies in view of the extent of labour and costs. While reviewing the effects of ACTH analogues on human performance (Gaillard, 1981), I was struck by the tendency to ignore the possibility of type I errors. In particular, when using test batteries, a large number of statistical tests are carried out, only a few of which turn out to be significant. For example, if there are 10 tests, each yielding a total of two scores (e.g., speed and accuracy), there is a total of 20 scores. Very little can be said if only two or three scores are significant, and the evidence is particularly weak in case of the usual practice of post-hoc interpretation: the value of a 'significant' effect is further undermined by using more than one statistical design for the same data set. Thus, in addition to analyses of variance, t-tests are carried out. Another common malpractice is to use both placebo vs. treatment comparisons and pre-post treatment comparisons on the same day and then to take the most 'reliable' result. Results are seldom replicated in human psychopharmacology. For instance, the above-mentioned ACTH review covered about 100 studies in which hardly any replications were reported. The task, the administration of the drug, the experimental design, and the type of subjects were changed so that comparisons between studies were difficult. Yet such changes are repeatedly used by authors as post-hoc explanations of why a particular drug effect was found in one but not another study. The possibility was never mentioned that the observed drug effect might in fact be a type I error implying that the drug had no real influence.

Concluding Remarks

There seems to be no generally agreed methodology in human psychopharmacology. One reason for this may be that several disciplines are involved each with different theoretical backgrounds and different research strategies. More research is necessary on the utility of the various study designs and the validity of tasks and procedures. The psychological significance is known for only a minority of the tasks used. In particular it is not known which mental processes are involved when batteries of tests are used. The practical validity of laboratory tasks has not been examined and future research must be planned to investigate the extent to which laboratory tasks predict task performance in everyday life.

References

Frowein HW (1981) *Selective Drug Effects on Information Processing*. Soesterberg: Monograph of the TNO Institute for Perception.

Frowein HW, Reitsma D and Acquariusc (1981) Effects of two counteracting stresses on the reaction process In: Baddeley AD and Long JL (eds.) *Attention and Performance IX*. Hillsdale, New Jersey: Erlbaum.

Gaillard AWK (1980) The use of task variables and brain potentials in the assessment of cognitive impairment in epileptic patients. In: Kulig BM, Meinardi H and Stores G (eds.) *Epilepsy and Behavior 1979*. pp. 104–110 Lisse: Swets and Zeitlinger.

Gaillard AWK (1981) ACTH analogs and human performance. In: Martinez JL Jr, Jensen RA, Messing RB, Rigter H and McGaugh JL (eds.) *Endogenous Peptides and Learning and Memory Processes*. pp. 181–196 New York: Academic Press.

Hockey GRJ, Gaillard AWK and Coles MGH (eds.) (1986) *Energetics and Human Information Processing*. Dordrecht: Martinus Nijhoff.

Poulton EC and Freeman PR (1966) Unwanted asymmetrical transfer effects with balanced experimental designs. *Psychol. Bull.* **66**, 1–8

Sanders AF (1980) Stage analysis of reaction processes. In: Stelmach G and Requin J (eds.) *Tutorials on Motor Behavior* Amsterdam: North-Holland.

Sanders AF (1983) Towards a model of stress and human performance. *Acta Psychol.* **53**, 61–97

Sternberg S (1969) On the discovery of processing stages: some extension of Donder's method. *Acta Psychol.* 30, 276–315.

Psychopharmacology and Reaction Time
Edited by I. Hindmarch, B. Aufdembrinke and H. Ott
© 1988 John Wiley & Sons Ltd

3

Two Experimental Approaches to Specifying Drug Effects: Physiological and Subjective State vs. Information Processing

G. Debus and S. Börgens

Institute of Psychology, RWTH, Aachen, FRG

Abstract

This paper outlines a comparison between two experimental approaches that aim at specifying the occurrence or relative size of drug effects. One is focused on information processing; its main dependent variable is reaction time. The other is focused on measuring physiological and subjective state. The two approaches have distinct theoretical and methodological backgrounds. Their common features and their differences are briefly discussed. In addition, their relative advantages and disadvantages with respect to reliability and generalization are outlined. A combination or even an integration of the approaches could be useful in the study of many research issues.

Introduction

The most common approach to specifying drug effects can be termed measure oriented. Measures that are thought to be pharmacosensitive are selected from the provinces of performance and subjective ratings or physiological states, e.g., reaction time, and autonomic arousal. This kind of research should be regarded with scepticism, since the results are often not replicable—presumably because different influences modify the effect of a drug. Such influences are often ignored for want of a suitable theoretical framework.

This measure orientation can be contrasted with an experimental orientation which specifies drug effects in terms of experimental variables that influence their occurrence or size in behavioural measures. This rationale provides greater reliability and generalizability because it describes drug effects in terms of basic organismic processes and states to the extent that they are under the control of experimental manipulations.

Within the experimental orientation, two approaches can be further distinguished: the first deals with changes of the subject's state, which may be indicated by physiological, subjective, and occasionally by performance measures. The second approach deals with changes of information processing investigated primarily by means of performance measures. The first approach is labelled state oriented, the second performance oriented.

Reaction time has a different function in the two approaches. While in the state-oriented approach it is a rather indirect index of state, it is a central indicator of information processing in the performance-oriented approach. Although both approaches claim to analyse the locus of drug action in psychological terms, each has its own theoretical background and tradition. The aim of this paper is to compare the relative merits and weaknesses of the two approaches in order to show how they might contribute to the localization of drug action.

General Outlines

To illustrate the two approaches, imagine two typical experimental situations in which drug effects can be studied. The first is typical of the state-oriented approach: a situation involving the anticipation of painful stimuli. Electrodes are attached to the subject, who is told that unpleasant but harmless electric shocks will be administered at regular intervals. The subject knows that a shock will be given each time a digital clock counting backwards from 10 to zero reaches zero. In the control condition, the subject anticipates the presentation of a coloured light. In the anticipation periods, various indices of anxiety and apprehension, such as ratings and physiological variables, are assessed.

The second situation is characteristic of the performance-oriented approach: a choice reaction task in which the subject sits in front of a square visual display with a target button at each corner. Before signal presentation, the subject rests his index finger on a release button. As soon as a geometric pattern appears pointing one of the four corners, the corresponding target button has to be pressed. Fitts (Fitts and Peterson, 1964) claims that two indices can be obtained: the time between stimulus onset and movement initiation (reaction time) and the time between initiation and completion of the movement (movement time). The application of the additive factor method (Sternberg, 1969; Sanders, 1980) suggests a variation of different aspects of the task. For example, the above condition of high stimulus–response compatibility can be compared with a condition of low stimulus–response compatibility, in which the task is to press the next button in a counter-clockwise direction rather than to press the adjacent button.

Comparison of the Approaches

The state- and performance-oriented approaches have various similarities as well as differences; these will now be briefly outlined.
The common features include the following:

1. The four major elements of both approaches are the same, i.e., theoretical constructs, dependent measures, experimental variations, and drugs. This is shown in Table 1 for our own research and that of Frowein (1981) as typical examples.
2. Both approaches aim at drawing conclusions about the loci of drug actions in terms of theoretical constructs.
3. In both approaches, experimental variables are selected which are theoretically or empirically considered relevant to certain theoretical constructs.
4. The experimental design is usually factorial, varying simultaneously situational and drug variables.
5. Statistical inference from such a design is usually based on the results of analyses of variance. If experimental variables interact, they are thought to affect a common process. If the effects are additive, the corresponding variables are thought to affect different processes. This is illustrated further in Figures 1 and 2.

Figure 1 is an idealized representation of two results of the state-oriented approach (Janke, 1964; Erdmann *et al.*, 1984). They show the effects of various drugs and different experimental variations thought to induce anxiety, and trait anxiety as a classification variable, upon variables such as skin

Table 1. Overview of constructs, measure, experimental conditions, and drugs in the state-oriented and the performance-oriented approach

Approach	STATE resp. STAGE	Measure	Conditions	Drugs
State-oriented	Anxiety	Hand steadiness Spontaneous skin responses Rating 'anxiety'	Trait anxiety Public speaking simulation Pain anticipation	Tranquilizers Sedatives Beta-blockers
Performance-oriented	Stimulus preprocessing Stimulus encoding Response selection Motor programming Response execution	Reaction time Movement time	Stimulus intensity Stimulus quality Stimulus–response Time on task Movement amplitude	Barbiturate Amphetamine

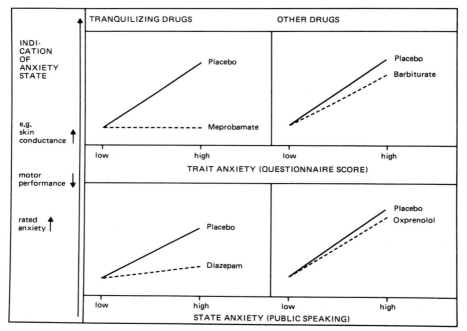

Figure 1. Idealized illustration of results of the state-oriented approach (*above:* Janke, 1964; *below:* Erdmann *et al.,* 1984; see text for further information).

resistance, anxiety ratings, and motor performance. Note that the downward direction in the figure always refers to tranquilizer-typical effects in the sense of reduced anxiety. It can be seen that minor tranquilizers such as meprobamate and diazepam tend to interact with experimental variations to produce beneficial effects compared with placebo in conditions that are supposed to increase anxiety, yet produce no such effects in neutral conditions. This pattern does not apply to beta-blockers. Thus, there seems to exist a mode of action typical for tranquilizers, possibly related to the development of anxiety.

Figure 2 shows a similar idealized picture of the main results of Frowein (1981). In a series of experiments, he varied task parameters which are believed to act selectively upon different stages of information processing. He found that a barbiturate interacted only with stimulus quality. This led to the conclusion that a barbiturate selectively affects the encoding stage of information processing. On the other hand, amphetamine only interacted with variables such as movement amplitude and time on task; and so Frowein concluded that amphetamine acts upon late stages of information processing concerned with motor control execution.

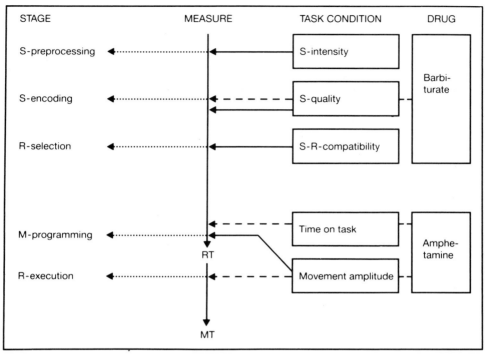

Figure 2. Idealized illustration of some main results of Frowein's work. *Solid lines* represent main effect. *Dashed lines* represent interactions of the two factors (drug/task condition). *Dotted lines* represent the inference from an effect upon the underlying processing stage. RT, reaction time; MT, movement time; S, stimulus; R, response; M, motor.

Differences

There are also differences between the approaches. First, there is a difference in the type of dependent variable. The state-oriented method is characterized by a multi-method approach. The choice of dependent variables of performance and subjective and physiological states is governed by a theoretical construct. Such a construct might be some mood state, such as anxiety, or a pattern of activation, such as increased arousal.

The performance-oriented method is concerned with clearly defined performance variables, namely, reaction time and, frequently, movement time. All information processing between stimulus onset and response initiation is supposed to follow a linear stage model. This means that each processing stage needs a certain amount of time. Reaction time reflects the total time required.

There are two points to be made with regard to the selection of experimental variables. There is a different logic behind the selection of experimental variations and the range of variation: the state-oriented approach derives operational definitions from a theoretical construct. The performance-oriented approach adopts a more inductive procedure (cf. Prinz, 1972), relying upon the results of preceding additive factor experiments to discover the processing stages.

As a consequence of these divergent rationales, the manipulations differ in complexity and selectivity. The state-oriented approach uses situations which differ in many aspects. Stress situations are used, e.g., noise, failure feedback, anticipation of painful stimuli, and public speaking. The performance-oriented approach uses variations which are closely connected with the task requirements, e.g., stimulus intensity and stimulus frequency. The two approaches could thus be labelled in terms macro- versus micro-manipulation of variables.

At first glance, inferences about the loci of drug action seem to differ in the two approaches: states in terms of specific moods (anxiety, anger) or energy resources (arousal) versus stages of information processing. The difference seems to vanish in the conceptualization of energy processing components relating to structural components (Sanders, 1983). The energetic components concern so-called functional variables such as accessory stimuli, time uncertainty, and time on task. If, furthermore, variables like time of day and sleep deprivation are included, the gap between the state-oriented and performance-oriented approach may be bridged.

The two approaches have also been applied differently in research: the state-oriented approach has been used in differential psychology, experimental psychology of emotion, and clinical psychopharmacology. In the former, drugs have been used to test hypotheses about sources of individual differences (Janke, 1983a). In research into emotion, drugs have been used to investigate the question of physiological patterns specific to an emotion (Erdmann, 1983; Janke *et al.*, 1986) or the relative influence of peripheral and central physiological states upon emotion formation. In clinical psychopharmacology, drugs have been tested in order to detect components of drug action, such as sedating components, and to predict therapeutic efficacy (Janke and Debus, 1975).

The performance-oriented approach has so far been guided by a theoretical interest in information processing (for a summary, see Callaway, 1983). Its main purpose has been to regard drugs as conditions which selectively affect distinct stages. Drugs are presumed to change the state of the organism. Hence, they are subsumed under the class of functional variables.

To summarize: we conclude that the two experimental approaches originate from quite different backgrounds. Only recently, ideas have been developed that allow the establishment of a manual communication.

Evaluation of the Two Approaches

Both approaches have certain advantages and disadvantages as far as internal validity is concerned. Some important points will now be discussed.

Experimental setting

Both approaches differ in the constraints they impose upon the subject's activity in a given situation or in a given task. In performance-oriented studies, we may assume that subjects are primarily occupied with the cognitive activity of task completion. This is a well-known assumption in linear stage models (Gopher and Sanders, 1984). In contrast, in the state-oriented approach, subjects can, within limits, react in different ways; these are termed 'changing strategies' and 'coping modes'. Suppose subjects have to speak in public (as an example of an anxiety-arousing condition): they can react in various ways. e.g., they can give themselves instructions, worry about the situation, prepare themselves for the speech. Thus, although the experimental variation is in both cases fixed and open to replication, the subjects' reactions in the latter case are much less determined and thus negatively influence internal validity.

Status of the dependent variables

Reaction time measures as used in the performance-oriented approach reflect information processing in real time. In the state-oriented approach, the variables are indices of a construct that is inaccessible to direct observation. The relation between the index and underlying construct is far from perfect. The internal validity of variables in the state-oriented approach therefore seems to be weaker than that of time measures.

Relationship between independent and dependent variables

With regard to interactions in the factorial experimental design, both approaches assume a linear relationship between independent and dependent variables. If this is not the case, spurious interactions may be produced that are then erroneously interpreted as functional convergences of the independent variables. The advantage of the performance-oriented approach is that, because it is restricted to clear-cut experimental variations, investigations can be more easily replicated with various ranges of the independent variable, and so the linearity of relations can be checked.

Logic of inference

Both approaches pose one major statistical problem. If two manipulations yield significant main effects but no significant interaction upon the dependent variable, they are thought to be independent and to act upon different processes. But there is no proper way of determining the risk of a type II error.

This problem can be crucial in the performance-oriented approach, where the absence of an interaction is seen positively as showing additivity, while the proponents of the state-oriented approach would, having expected a significant interaction, wonder why it failed to occur and so replicate or modify the experiment. Thus, the risk of a type II error seems to be somewhat slighter in the state-oriented approach.

Furthermore, one should emphasize the arguments against the notion that the additive factor method is a suitable tool for generating a theory just by sophisticated data analysis (Prinz, 1972). Making inferences from additive effects at different processing stages is unwarranted unless appropriate theoretical considerations are made.

Quality of psychometric data

A final advantage of the performance-oriented approach is the quality of its psychometric data. Chronometric measures conform to a ratio scale. For the state-oriented approach, the picture is at best mixed. While most physiological measures, e.g., heart rate, number of spontaneous skin conductance responses, and body temperature, conform to an interval or ratio scale, the quality of psychometric ratings of subjective state may even fail to reach interval level, making parametric tests such as analyses of variance seem unwarranted.

In summary, the performance-oriented approach has reasonable advantages as far as internal validity is concerned. With regard to generalizability or external validity, the following comparisons can be made.

Diversity of measures

The fact that conclusions from state-oriented studies are based on different kinds of measures suggests at first glance that they have more general applicability. Unfortunately, there is little empirical evidence that drug responses apply generally to different measures, even if they deal with the same construct (Janke, 1983b). Dissociations between objective and subjective measures are not uncommon; and care should be taken not to overestimate the potential for generalizations. On the other hand, the possibilities for making generalizations from results of choice reaction time tasks of the performance-related approach should not be underestimated. The rationale behind this second approach is to obtain information about basic components of information processing, structural energetic, and then to generalize on that basis. Frowein's studies, for instance, are a good example of the potential external validity of this approach; his results are in accordance with quite different experiments using other measures.

It can be concluded that both approaches derive their measures from certain theoretical constructs. Inasmuch as drug effects are specified on the basis of these constructs, the two approaches are basically equivalent as far as generalizations are concerned. But since the state-oriented approach uses more general constructs, its potential for making generalizations may be greater.

Situational and task variables

Similar conclusions can be drawn with regard to the generalization of drug responses in different situations and tasks. Again, the state-oriented approach should not be overestimated. Drug responses in situations which are thought to be specific emotion-inducing conditions, e.g., for anxiety, public speaking, or anticipation of pain (cf. Janke 1983b), differ in many aspects. Obviously, a particular kind of drug response is more probable in one construct-related type of situation than in another. There is evidence, for example, that tranquilizers stabilize emotions in anxiety states, yet have no such effect or even a paradoxical effect in emotionally neutral states.

Limits to generalizations become evident when situations do not tap the inherent construct of a particular approach. For example, how can we generalize from results of performance tests so as to be pertinent to anxiety states? This is only conceivable if anxiety is defined in terms of energy resources such as arousal. But there is no rationale for making generalizations if anxiety is defined as a specific emotional state and if a drug is seen as specifically affecting that state.

But it is doubtful whether results from a given task—with the limitations imposed upon energetic and structural components—can be generalized to a variety of tasks without changing the entire architecture of the processes involved. This applies particularly to the performance-oriented approach.

Subjects

The state-oriented approach takes into account inter-individual differences of personality traits. They are regarded as stable characteristics which permit more reliable predictions about the emotional state in a given situation. The generalization of drug effects therefore leads to differential predictions. In contrast, individual differences are largely ignored in studies of the performance-oriented approach.

So far, the state-oriented approach seems better prepared for dealing with different populations. This is especially true when predicting symptom- or syndrome-specific drug actions in patients.

The discussion of generalizations or external validity can be summarized as follows: the state-oriented approach has certain advantages due to its multi-method, multi-situation, and multi-subject experimentation, although in practice attempts towards generalization have not been very successful.

Both approaches are primarily analytical; hence, generalization to other measures, situations, tasks, and subjects is only feasible if more effort is devoted to construct validation of standard conditions.

Conclusions

We can conclude from the above discussion that the two approaches can be combined:

Integration.
To some extent, it may be possible to integrate the two approaches. Thus, individual differences in a subject's state at the time of performance might be changed by manipulating personality traits and situational conditions. Such manipulations must, of course, be based on definite hypotheses about the site of drug action. The addition of trait and situational variables to task variables and the analysis of their effects upon a dependent variable, such as reaction time, would augment our knowledge about how drugs operate in actual behaviour.

For example, the improvement of motor performance that is frequently observed in anxious patients under the influence of a tranquilizer could be used to predict the outcome of an experiment in an integrated framework. One could expect an interaction between tranquilizer, trait or state anxiety, and task variables that affect the processing stages controlling motor preparation and execution.

Predictions about the alternative approach.
Even if an integration of the two approaches seems inappropriate, it may still be possible to predict the outcome of the alternative approach.

For example, in an attempt to explain individual differences of response to tranquilizers, Janke and Debus (1972) proposed two components of drug action. The first component was sedative; the second concerned emotional stability. If this inference is valid, one might assume two different sites of drug action: one in the encoding stage and one in the stages of motor programming and execution. Thus, task variables such as stimulus quality and target width could be the critical variables which have to be manipulated in a choice reaction task. Predictions in the reverse direction are also conceivable.

Complementarity.
The two approaches can complement each other. Both can be regarded as

restricted to a certain field of application. In that case, they will answer their own specific questions separately.

For example, according to Frowein (1981), a barbiturate selectively affects the encoding stage. It is well known that barbiturates also alleviate anxiety. As long as there is no unifying theoretical link between these two results, we have to adopt both approaches to derive information about different aspects of drug action.

The general conclusion of this discussion is that if the two approaches could be combined to yield convergent results and conclusions, then the internal and, hopefully, external validity of experimentation with drugs could be enhanced.

References

Callaway E (1983) The pharmacology of human information processing. *Psychophysiology* **20**, 359–70.

Erdmann G (1983) *Zur Beeinflußbarkeit emotionaler Prozesse durch vegetative Variation*. Weinheim: Beltz.

Erdmann G, Janke W, Köchers S and Terschlüsen B (1984) Comparison of the emotional effects of a beta-adrenergic blocking agent and a tranquilizer under different situational conditions. I. Anxiety-arousing situation. *Neuropshychobiology* **12**, 143–51.

Fitts P and Peterson JR (1964) Information capacity of discrete motor responses. *J. Exp. Psychol.* **67**, 103–12.

Frowein HW (1981) *Selective Drug Effects on Information Processing*. Soesterberg: Institute of Perception TNO.

Gopher D and Sanders AF (1984) S-Oh-R: Oh Stages! Oh Resources! In: Prinz W and Sanders AF (eds.) *Cognition and Motor Processes*. Berlin: Springer.

Janke W (1964) *Experimentelle Untersuchungen zur Abhängigkeit der Wirkung psychotroper Substanzen von Persönlichkeitsmerkmalen. Ein Beitrag zur Begründung einer differentiellen Pharmakophychologie*. Frankfurt: Akademische Verlagsgesellschaft.

Janke W (ed.) (1983a) *Response Variability to Psychotropic Drugs*. Oxford: Pergamon Press.

Janke W (1983b) Response variability to psychotropic drugs. Overview of the main approaches to differential pharmacopsychology. In: Janke W (ed.) *Response Variability to Psychotropic Drugs*. Oxford: Pergamon Press.

Janke W and Debus G (1972) Double-blind psychometric evaluation of pimozide and haloperidol versus placebo in emotionally labile volunteers under two different work load conditions. *Pharmakopsychiatrie, Neuro-Psychopharmakologie* **5**, 33–51.

Janke W and Debus G (1975) Pharmakopsychologische Untersuchungen an gesunden Probanden zur Prognose der therapeutischen Effizienz von Psychopharmaka. *Arzneimittelforschung* **25**, 1185–94.

Janke W, Debus G and Erdmann G (1986) Angstreduzierende Wirkung von Psychopharmaka bei gesunden Personen. Überblick über Ergebnisse experimenteller Untersuchungen und Schlußfolgerungen zur Bedeutung des Probandenversuchs zur Prädiktion anxiolytischer Wirkungen bei Patienten mit Angstsyndromen. In: Keupp W und Saletu B (eds.) *Biologische Psychiatrie*. Heidelberg: Springer.

Prinz W (1972). Reaktionszeit-Franktionierung durch Varianzanalyse? *Arch. Psychol.*
   124, 240–52
Sanders AF (1980) Stage analysis of reaction processes. In: Stelmach GE and Requin J
   (eds.) *Tutorials in Motor Behavior*. Amsterdam: North-Holland.
Sanders AF (1983) Towards a model of stress and human performance. *Acta Psychol.*
   53, 61–97.
Sternberg S (1969) On the discovery of processing stages: some extension of Donder's
   methods. *Acta Psychol.* **30**, 279–315.

Psychopharmacology and Reaction Time
Edited by I. Hindmarch, B. Aufdembrinke and H. Ott
© 1988 John Wiley & Sons Ltd

4

Age-related Visual Information Processing in Tasks of Different Complexity: A Concise Review

J. Beringer[1], J. Wandmacher[1], and R. Görtelmeyer[2]

[1]*Institute of Psychology, Technical University, Darmstadt, FRG.*
[2]*Clinical Research Department, E. Merck, Darmstadt, FRG.*

Abstract

A study of various investigations of ageing suggests that there is one general slowing mechanism within the information processing system. The relation between the latencies of old and young subjects can be described by one general function (the age function), reflecting a proportional slowing of all cognitive processes. Some of the available evidence is briefly summarized. It is suggested that automatic processes may be an exception to the rule, although current notions of attention and automaticity seem to be at odds with this possibility.

Introduction

Today's research into age-dependent changes in the speed of information processing is greatly influenced by the idea that the flow of information in the human system can be divided into sequential steps. This notion of steps or processing stages has provided a new theoretical framework and new objectives to research into behavioural effects of slowing with age (Birren *et al.*, 1980). Many experiments have been carried out with the aim of locating the slowing phenomenon in specific processing stages. The idea has been to use various experimental variables which are known to affect different stages and to find an interaction with age only in some critical stages. Age-dependent deficits have, however, been obtained with almost all tasks and this must be interpreted as evidence for a general slowing of the information processing system (Birren *et al.*, 1980; Hoyer and Plude, 1980).

That performance deficits in different stages seem to be related to each other suggests that the slowing of processing is caused by one general mechanism. According to the complexity hypothesis of Cerella *et al.* (1980), the magnitude of age effects on reaction times is proportional to the difficulty or complexity of the task. The ratio of the reaction time of old subjects to that of young subjects should therefore remain fairly constant across different levels of task

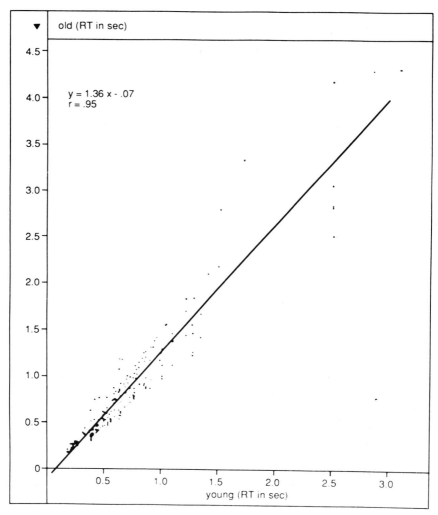

Figure 1. Age function and mean reaction times of young and old subjects in 99 different tasks. (From Cerella *et al.,* 1980. © 1980 by the American Psychological Association. Reprinted by permission of the publisher and author.)

complexity (Lindholm and Parkinson, 1983). Similarly, the reaction time of old subjects should be a linear function of the reaction time of young subjects with a slope greater than unity. This function will be called the age function. The amount of variance which is explained when predicting reaction times of old subjects by means of the age function provides evidence for or against the complexity hypothesis. The age function usually explains more than 90% of the variance of the reaction time of old subjects (Cerella *et al.*, 1980). The slope amounts to 1.36, and the intercept is about zero (see Figure 1).

A linear age-function suggests that with advanced age virtually all processing stages are affected by the same factor (Salthouse and Somberg, 1982). Green (1983) has pointed out that such general linear models as the age function can be generalized to dynamic models which consider age as a continuous variable. These age dynamic models predict that speed of processing will exponentially decline with age. This could mean that age-related slowing is caused by a random decay process of the neuronal connections because in that case one would expect an exponential dynamic component (Green, 1983).

The application of the age function to the analysis of response latencies has direct implications for the traditional way of interpreting interaction effects. A significant interaction between age and task complexity does not necessarily reflect a specific deficit. If the age effect is proportional to task complexity—defined in terms of the reaction time of young subjects—there is evidence for one general slowing factor in the entire information processing system of older subjects rather than for a specific deficit (Lindholm and Parkinson, 1983; Salthouse and Somberg, 1982). A brief review of some typical age comparisons will demonstrate how useful the application of an age function can be for interpreting interaction effects.

Evidence for the Complexity Hypothesis

The most clear-cut evidence in favour of the complexity hypothesis within a single experiment and across different processing stages is provided by Salthouse and Somberg (1982). Old and young subjects (each n = 24) performed a Sternberg memory search task with digits. Task complexity was varied within three different stages: the encoding stage (degradation pattern), the comparison stage (memory set size), and the response choice stage (yes–no response vs. digit response). Salthouse and Somberg found significant interactions between age and each of the three complexity interactions between age and each of the three complexity factors. The difference in reaction time between old and young subjects increased proportionately with task complexity. This is reflected by the parameters of the estimated age function: 2.16 for the slope and 0.31 for the intercept (explained variance 96%).

Salthouse and Somberg concluded that although there are significant interaction effects, there is apparently no age difference specifically related to a particular processing stage. Rather, the multiplicative relationship suggests an age-associated slowing that is dependent on the amount of central processing required in a given task.

Evidence for the complexity hypothesis within a single experiment was also found in a letter-matching task by Lindholm and Parkinson (1983). They used four different complexity levels: simple reaction time (RT), choice RT, physical match (PM), and name match (NM) to realize different levels of encoding complexity: simple < choice < PM < NM. The experiment was run with a sample of 16 subjects for each age group. The stimulus set consisted of the upper and lower case letters A, H, T, F. The ranking of the difference in response latencies relating to the levels of processing complexity was observed. The interaction between complexity and age was also significant. The assumption of a constant relative age difference was tested by a logarithmic transformation of the reaction time, because constant reaction time ratios become equal differences on a logarithmic scale. The significant interaction between complexity and age should therefore disappear for the logarithms of the reaction times.

While this prediction held for the first three complexity levels, there remained a significant interaction when the name identity task (NM) was included. Lindholm and Parkinson located the origin of this inconsistency in a subset of stimuli within the naming task. Old subjects had disproportionate difficulties in classifying the physically similar letters 't' and 'f' as not being name identical. Despite this inconsistency, their results were interpreted as evidence for a general age-related reduction of processing speed. They argued that if there was a specific age-associated deficit in retrieving letter names, the response times of the old subjects should have been disproportionately long for all of the letter pairs. Yet a linear age function with a slope of 1.63 and an intercept of -79.17 described the whole set of data quite well ($r = 0.99$) even with 't' and 'f' included.

Nevertheless, the complexity hypothesis might be inadequate for variations in complexity due to the physical similarity of the stimulus material. If processing in the encoding stage of old subjects is not only slowed but also more noisy, a qualitative difference may arise due to data limitation which can only be compensated for by additional processing in order to perform accurately. Thus, confusing stimulus material is likely to produce disproportionate effects with age. In the same way, masking may also produce disproportionate demands on processing, provided that old subjects encode less input and continue processing on less information than young subjects. The results of Walsh (1982) and Cerella *et al.* (1982) on age-dependent backward masking support this view, because proportionate slowing effects were not obtained in either case. In the study of Cerella *et al.* (1982) this limitation even forced subjects to change their way of processing.

Apart from situations relating to information acquisition, the complexity hypothesis may also fail in some other situations. When a subject performs a task, the task-imposed degrees of freedom determine how accurately the results may reflect invariant characteristics, such as slowing of the processing systems. This means that studies which are concerned with differences in processing strategies (Cohen and Faulkner, 1983) cannot be interpreted in terms of complexity hypothesis. Thus, differences in preparation strategies can produce a disproportionate loss of speed in old subjects as Rabbitt (1979) has demonstrated with regard to age-dependent repetition effects. If, however, the repetition effect is controlled by partially valid cues, the age-related slowing is again proportionate (Madden, 1984). It might be that the cueing technique provided more control over the preparation strategies of both age groups in successive trials.

The review of these studies demonstrates that although the age function cannot be applied to all paradigms, this method of analysis clearly adds to the understanding of the interaction between age and task (Cerella *et al.*, 1980).

There are also a few experiments of ageing which are not concerned with stage of processing but with the issue of automatic vs. controlled processing. These studies provide evidence against a general slowing concept (Farkas and Hoyer, 1980; Plude and Hoyer, 1981). Thus, automatic processes seem to slow down less with age than controlled processes (Schneider *et al.*, 1984). This finding agrees with resource notions of attention (Wickens, 1984) which ascribe age-related speed decrements to a general capacity limitation in older subjects (Craik and Byrd, 1982; Farkas and Hoyer, 1980; Hasher and Zacks, 1979; Plude and Hoyer, 1981). If this were valid, one should expect no; or at least a smaller; speed difference in automatic processes because these are considered capacity free. This line of reasoning, however, depends on the interpretation of the concept of attention. The success of resource notions as a conceptual framework for research in attention can be questioned (Allport, 1980; Neumann, 1984a). Various notions of attention will therefore be outlined before the age-related phenomena are discussed.

Concepts of Attention

Besides the resource theories, there are so-called structural theories of attention. Structural theories are primarily concerned with the locus, or loci, of processing limitations within the processing system under the assumption that external information is initially processed in parallel. At some level processing becomes serial, capacity limited and controlled. Depending on the proposed locus of processing limitations the theories are called early (Treisman and

Gelade, 1980) or late selection (Duncan, 1980; Schneider and Shiffrin, 1977).

Early selection proposes that parallel processing is limited to simple sensory features. Even the conjunction of separable features would require serial processing through focusing attention (Treisman and Gelade, 1980). In contrast, late selection theories claim that inputs are processed in parallel up to a semantic level of encoding and that only the response selection stage constitutes a bottleneck (Duncan, 1980).

Parallel visual search on the basis of category membership of a target (Schneider and Shiffrin, 1977) or unavoidable extraction of word meaning in a Stroop situation are classic examples in favour of late selection. Recently, however, these results have been questioned because the category effect seems to be strongly dependent on the degree of physical similarity within the stimulus set (Duncan, 1983; Krueger, 1984; Mohr, 1984), and the Stroop effect depends on the spatial configuration of word and colour (Francolini and Egeth, 1980; Kahneman and Henik, 1981). Elements of early selection therefore appear to play a role in classic examples of late selection tasks.

Neither resource nor structural theories provide a satisfactory set of explanations for the entire range of empirical data. One solution might be to consider capacity limitations of the human processing system in terms of a functional constraint as a consequence of the need to converge the entire sensory input to just one action (Kahneman and Treisman, 1984; Neumann, 1984b). From this point of view, the limits of parallel processing depend on the combination of the actual stimulus situation and the required action. Instead of attempts to locate structural bottlenecks in certain processing stages, one should rather attempt to formulate conditions in which bottlenecks occur as a consequence of functional constraints.

The level of control (Neumann, 1984b) approach might be helpful in describing such conditions. In terms of this approach, an action can only be executed when sufficient variables for controlling the action are specified 'A process becomes automatic, if its parameters are sufficiently specified by a skill in conjunction with input information' (Neumann). According to LaBerge (1981), typical mechanisms of skill development in visual search are unification and association of representation codes.

Schneider (1985) has stressed this alternative view by formulating a communication theory of attention. In analogy to communication networks, the human processing system consists of communication channels in which successive layers of nodes converge. In case of multiple input information interference arises at converging nodes causing the loss of all but the strongest information. The gain in conjunction with the input characteristics of each channel determines what information will be transmitted. In terms of this theory, the question is no longer whether it is possible to process sensory input in a parallel or serial mode but rather which mode is the most effective. This point of view has the advantage of breaking the dichotomy of early and late selection by emphasizing the great importance of the input constellation in determining whether parallel or serial processing is more effective. Thus, factors such as spatial grouping (Kahneman and Henik, 1981), colour (Francolini and Egeth, 1980), and possibly even object identity (Kahneman and Treisman, 1984) appear to influence the mode of processing in a given task.

In the context of a functional approach, automaticity of an action reduces cognitive processing demands in that more variables of the desired action are specified in advance and that information pick-up skills are restructured and optimized (Cheng, 1985). This means that there are no *a priori* reasons why age-related effects on performance in tasks with varying attentional demands should differ from effects on other tasks with varying complexity. The complexity hypothesis (Cerella *et al.*, 1980) should also hold when attentional demands change.

Age-related Effects on Visual Attention

In a card-sorting paradigm, Rabbitt (1965) investigated the effect of age on performance in visual search. He obtained a significant interaction between the effects of display size (1, 2, 5, 9 simultaneous items) and age, and between the effects of target size, display set size, and age. In Figure 2 Rabbitt's data are rearranged as an age function with parameter values of 1.32 for the slope and 4.62 for the intercept. (All age functions were estimated by determining the first principal component with the least squares method.) It appears that age-dependent performance on this type of search with varying display and target set sizes can roughly be fitted by a linear function with a slope value comparable to that of the earlier described age functions.

Wright and Elias (1979) studied the effect of age on performance in visual filtering. Subjects attended to one target that was always displayed at the same position. The target was flanked by a pair of irrelevant letters which were to be completely ignored. There were four conditions: a) target without flanking letters, b) target with response irrelevant letters, c) target with response consistent letters, d) target with response inconsistent letters. In view of results from Stroop experiments, Wright and Elias (1979) expected stronger interference of the flanking letters with old subjects. Yet the results showed that old and young subjects were about equally affected by response irrelevant letters, that old subjects profited less from a response consistent context, and that old subjects were less affected by a response inconsistent context. Thus, less positive and less negative interference was observed in the old subjects than in the young subjects. Wright and Elias assumed that if young subjects adapt a strategy to respond on the mere basis of physical features—without completing the full target analysis—they should be generally faster and be more affected by inconsistent context than old subjects. A trade-off between

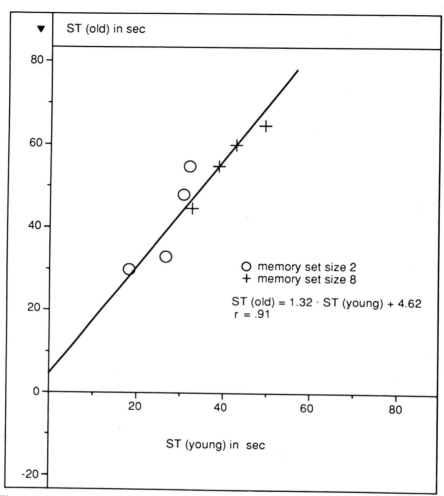

Figure 2. Estimated age function and mean sorting times of young and old subjects on a visual search experiment; from Rabbit, 1985.

processing speed and amount of interference would obviously overrule a simple proportional relation between response latencies as a function of task complexity. The results indeed show that estimates of the age function in the no context and in the neutral context conditions delivered reasonable linear parameter values ($b = 1.20$ and $a = 0.576$) while the two interference conditions systematically deviated from linearity.

Early selection was investigated by Farkas and Hoyer (1980) both in visual filtering and in visual search. They wondered whether young, middle-aged, and old subjects might differ in the use of spatial orientation of search items.

Their target stimulus was similar to a letter 'T' except that there was a short line segment on both ends of the long line segment. Their three conditions were a) target only, b) target with three distractor stimuli contrasting in the orientation of the longer line segment (horizontal vs. vertical), and c) target with three distractor stimuli that did not differ in orientation.

In the search task, the target could be located at each of four positions. contrasting and similar distractors slowed the old subjects but not the middle-aged or young subjects, suggesting an 'age-related deficit in the efficiency of the relatively automatic search process which operates when stimulus differences act to segregate task-relevant from task-irrelevant information' (Farkas and Hoyer, 1980). While this interpretation is statistically correct, estimates of the age function show that the slowing of old subjects was still proportional to the slowing of young subjects. The age function relating old to young subjects had the parameters $b = 2.73$ and $a = -8.0$ ($r = 0.99$). The corresponding parameters for the relation between middle-aged to young subjects were $b = 1.41$ and $a = -2.5$ ($r = 0.99$).

With exactly the same stimulus material Farkas and Hoyer (1980) performed a filtering experiment in which the position of the target was always the same and known in advance. Old subjects were considerably slower in the noncontrasting context condition, while young subjects were virtually unaffected. Farkas and Hoyer postulated a new age-related deficit, namely the 'difficulty of imposing perceptual organization on an array when task-relevant information is not differentiated from task-irrelevant information by stimulus factors'. Although the estimated age function fits quite well ($r = 0.99$), the slope, $b = 7.71$, is so high that indeed one cannot consider this result as proportional slowing. Middle-aged subjects were slowed with the usual ratio of $b = 1.41$ and intercept $a = -17.1$.

Yet before accepting a special age-related deficit, one should consider the possibility that the extremely high slowing ratio is stimulus specific. The crucial feature discriminating between target and distractor was the additional short line segment on the 'T' figure. This line was only 2.5 mm long, and in the case of a context with the same orientation the short line segment of the distractor adjacent to the target was quite close to the target. Thus, not only orientation but also physical closeness of the discriminating features might have caused the disproportionate decrement in performance. As outlined above, disproportionately long sorting times are likely to occur with old subjects using 'confusable' stimulus material.

Taken together, the results of serial visual search and filtering tasks fit well with the hypothesis of a general age-related slowing of mental processes. The results which are inconsistent with the age function can be readily attributed to methodological deficits.

Madden and Nebes (1980) trained old and young subjects in nine sessions in a consistent mapping condition to compare the development of automatic

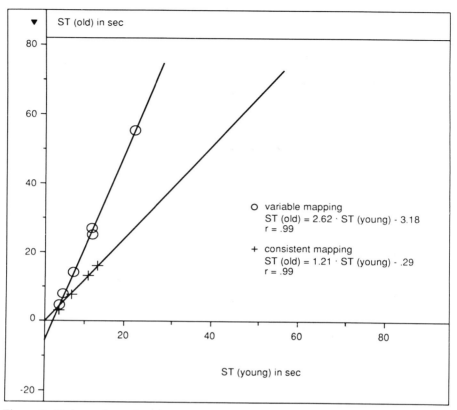

Figure 3. Estimated age function and mean sorting times for two mapping conditions from a visual search study; from Plude and Hoyer, 1981.

processes in both age samples. Eight old and eight young subjects searched for letter targets among letter distractors. The development of parallel search was indicated by the slope of the function relating search time to three different memory set sizes (1, 2, 3) see Schneider and Fisk, 1982.

Madden and Nebes found a significant interaction between the effects of age and memory set size. The latter effect was larger for old subjects, but as practice increased the set size effect decreased at an identical rate for both age groups. Moreover, the ratio between the reaction times of young and old subjects was constant across the different memory set sizes. Thus, the development of automatic components during search does not seem to be affected by age. The parameters of the corresponding age function averaged across the nine sessions were 1.83 for the slope and -166.8 for the intercept ($r = 0.99$). Since Madden and Nebes's visual search task certainly included automatic components, it is apparent that the age function could be applied to automatic processes.

Yet more definitive information might come from a study in which automatic and controlled search are realized within a single experiment. This is what Plude and Hoyer (1981) did in a card-sorting paradigm. In six sessions, eight subjects from each age group sorted cards, searching for targets among distractors with display sizes of 1, 4, and 9 items and memory set sizes of 2 and 4 targets. Subjects were divided into a consistent mapping and a variable mapping group. In variable mapping, older subjects slowed down significantly more than young subjects as display and memory set size increased, but in consistent mapping, there was no significant difference between both age groups. Indeed age function estimates for each mapping condition differ considerably in slope values (see Figure 3). The linear function for consistent mapping has the parameters $b = 1.21$ and $a = -0.3$, and the function for variable mapping shows $b = 2.62$ and $a = -3.2$. This is in contradiction to the complexity hypothesis of Cerella *et al.* (1980), which proposes only one general slowing factor. The results instead suggest separate slowing mechanisms for controlled and automatic processing (Hoyer and Plude, 1980); Plude and Hoyer, 1981; Davies *et al.*, 1984).

The investigations of Plude and Hoyer (1981), however, could have some methodological problems limiting the ultimate scope of the result. First, the most interesting factor, automatic vs. controlled search (consistent vs. variable mapping), was varied between subjects. Second, for each age and mapping condition, there were only four subjects in each group, which is insufficient for a conclusive interpretation of the difference in slope between the age functions. Third, a card-sorting paradigm has inherent problems in realizing a variable mapping condition as defined by Schneider and Shiffrin (1977). For example, the variable target remained constant while sorting a deck of 37 cards, making the variable target in fact consistent within one deck. The speed of adapting to the defined target set within one deck might be slowed with increased age, thus causing a steeper slope of the age function in the variable condition. Plude and Hoyer's (1981) experiment does not seem to prove adequately that automatic processes are less slowed with age than controlled processes.

Conclusion

The review of various studies of age-related visual information processing favours the complexity hypothesis of Cerella *et al.* (1980). The role of automatic processes is neither supported by experimental evidence nor by theoretical notions. Although automatic processes might slow down less in terms of absolute amount, there is no reason to consider them to be an exception.

Some studies indicate that the appropriateness of the complexity hypothesis is limited. Generally, proportional age-related slowing will only be found in experimental data when

1. old subjects use the same processing (Cohen and Faulkner, 1983; Wright and Elias, 1979) or preparation strategy (Madden, 1984; Rabbitt, 1979);
2. old subjects are not forced to resort to additional processing in order to compensate limitations of information acquisition (Cerella *et al.*, 1982) in cases where young subjects do not suffer from similar limits;
3. old subjects work on the same sensory input information as young subjects (Farkas and Hoyer, 1980; Lindholm and Parkinson 1983).

It should be noted that the meaning of the parameters of the age function is not yet fully clear. Hence, the age function needs further mathematical and theoretical clarification. In particular, the intercept of the age function should be interpreted with caution. The age function should also not be extrapolated below the observed range of data, because reaction times of both age groups cannot become arbitrarily small. The lower end of the age function is determined by a theoretical minimum reaction time for each group, which in turn is determined by the time taken by peripheral processes independent of the treatment. A negative intercept is expected when these peripheral processes are less impaired with age than the central ones. Thus, a negative intercept is no indicator for or against the validity of the age function. Age functions of corrected reaction times are expected to cross the origin because much of the peripheral components should have been eliminated by subtraction of a baseline. When assuming that peripheral processes of old subjects are never faster than the corresponding processes of younger subjects, one possible estimate for the lower end of the age function is the point where both age groups would have the same latencies (lower end $= a/[1 - b]$).

Despite the caveats mentioned above, the complexity hypothesis should be considered as a useful heuristic model for studying age-related decrements of cognitive processes. Changes of its parameters, in particular of its slope, may provide interesting information about differences between populations and between treatments.

References

Allport DA (1980) Attention and performance. In: Claxton G, (ed.) *Cognitive Psychology—New Directions*. London: Routledge & Kegan Paul.

Birren JE, Woods AM and Williams MV (1980). Behavioral slowing with age: Causes, organisation, and consequences. In: Poon LW (ed.) *Aging in the 1980s: Psychological Issues*. Washington D.C: American Psychological Association.

Cerella J, Poon LW and Williams DM (1980) Age and the complexity hypothesis. In: Poon LW (ed.) *Aging in the 1980s: Psychological Issues*. Washington D.C: American Psychological Association.

Cerella J, Poon LW and Fozard JL (1982) Age and iconic read-out. *J. Gerontol.* **37**, 197–202.

Cheng PW (1985) Restructuring versus automaticity: Alternative accounts of skill acquisition. *Psychol. Rev.* **92**, 414–23.

Cohen G and Faulkner D (1983) Age differences in performance on two information-processing tasks: Strategy selection and processing efficiency. *J. Gerontol.* **38**, 447–54

Craik FIM and Byrd M (1982) Aging and cognitive deficits: The role of attentional resources. In: Craik FIM and Trehub S (eds.) *Aging and Cognitive Processes.* New York: Plenum Press.

Davies DR, Jones DM and Taylor A (1984) Selective and sustained attention tasks: Individual and group differences. In: Parasuraman R and Davies DR (eds.) *Varieties of Attention.* New York: Academic Press Inc.

Duncan J (1980) The locus of interference in the perception of simultaneous stimuli. *Psychol. Rev.* **87**, 272–300.

Duncan J (1983) Category effects in visual search: A failure to replicate the 'oh-zero' phenomenon. *Percept. Psychophysics* **34**, 221–32.

Farkas MS and Hoyer WJ (1980) Processing consequences of perceptual grouping in selective attention. *J. Gerontol.* **35**, 207–16.

Francolini CM and Egeth HE (1980) On the nonautomaticity of 'automatic' activation: Evidence of selective seeing. *Percep. Psychophysics* **27**, 331–42.

Green VL (1983) Age dynamic models of information processing task latency: A theoretical note. *J. Gerontol.* **38**, 46–50.

Hasher L and Zacks RT (1979) Automatic and effortful processes in memory. *J. Exp. Psychol. Gen.* **108**, 356–88.

Hoyer WJ and Plude DJ (1980) Attentional and perceptual processes in the study of cognitive aging. In: Poon LW (ed.) *Aging in the 1980s: Psychological Issues.* Washington D.C: American Psychological Association.

Kahnemann D and Henik A (1981) Perceptual organization and attention. In: Kubovy M and Pomeranz JR (eds.) *Perceptual Organization.* Hillsdale, New Jersey: Erlbaum.

Kahnemann D and Treisman A (1984) Changing views of attention and automaticity. In: Parasuraman R and Davies DR (eds.) *Varieties of Attention.* New York: Academic Press Inc.

Krueger LE (1984) The category effect in visual search depends on physical rather than conceptual differences. *Percept. Psychophysics* **35**, 558–64.

LaBerge D (1981) Automatic information processing: A review. In: Long J and Baddeley A (eds.) *Attention and Performance IX.* Hillsdale, New Jersey: Erlbaum.

Lindholm JM and Parkinson SR (1983) An interpretation of age-related differences in letter-matching performance. *Percept. Psychophysics* **33**, 283–94.

Madden DJ (1984) Data-driven and memory-driven selective attention in visual search. *J. Gerontol.* **39**, 72–8.

Madden DJ and Nebes D (1980) Aging and the development of automaticity in visual search. *Developmental Psychol.* **16**, 377–84.

Mohr W (1984) *Visuelle Wahrnehmung und Zeichenfunktion: Untersuchungen zur Grundlage des Kategorieneffekts bei der Wahrnehmung von Buchstaben und Ziffern.* Regensburg: Roderer.

Neumann O (1984a) Die Hypothese begrenzter Kapazität und die Funktion der Aufmerksamkeit. In: Neumann O (ed.) *Perspektiven der Kognitionspsychologie.* Heidelberg: Springer.

Neumann O (1984b) Automatic processing: A review of recent findings and a plea for an old theory. In: Prinz W and Sanders AF (eds.) *Cognition and Motor Processes.* Heidelberg: Springer.

Plude DJ and Hoyer WJ (1981) Adult age differences in visual search as a function of stimulus mapping and processing load. *J. Gerontol.* **36**, 598–604.

Rabbitt P (1965) An age-decrement in the ability to ignore irrelevant information. *J. Gerontol.* **20**, 233–8.

Rabbitt P (1979) Some experiments and a model for changes in attentional selectivity with old age. In: Hoffmeister F and Müller L (eds.) *Brain Functions in Old Age.* Berlin: Springer.

Salthouse TA and Somberg BL (1982) Isolating the age deficit in speeded performance. *J. Gerontol.* **37**, 59–63.

Schneider W (1985) Toward a model of attention and the development of automaticity. In: Posner M and Marin OS (eds.) *Attention and Performance XI.* Hillsdale, New Jersey: Erlbaum.

Schneider W, Dumais ST and Shiffrin RM (1984) Automatic and control processing and attention. In: Parasuraman R and Davies DR (eds.) *Varieties of Attention.* New York: Academic Press Inc.

Schneider W and Fisk AD (1982) Degree of consistent training: Improvements in search performance and automatic process development. *Percep. Psychophysics* **31**, 160–8.

Schneider W and Shiffrin RM (1977) Controlled and automatic human processing: I. Detection, search, and attention. *Psychol. Rev.* **84**, 1–66.

Treisman AM and Gelade G (1980) A feature-integration theory of attention. *Cognitive Psychol.* **12**, 97–136.

Walsh DA (1982) The development of visual information process in adulthood and old age. In: Craik FIM and Trehub S (eds.) *Aging and Cognitive Processes.* New York: Plenum Press.

Wickens CD (1984) Processing resources in attention. In: Parasuraman R and Davies DR (eds.) *Varieties of Attention.* New York: Academic Press Inc.

Wright LL and Elias JW (1979) Age differences in the effect of perceptual noise. *J. Gerontol.* **34**, 704–8.

Psychopharmacology and Reaction Time
Edited by I. Hindmarch, B. Aufdembrinke and H. Ott
© 1988 John Wiley & Sons Ltd

5

Age-related Automatic Versus Controlled Visual Search

J. Beringer[1], *J. Wandmacher*[1], *and R. Görtelmeyer*[2]

[1]*Institute of Psychology, Technical University, Darmstadt, FRG.*
[2]*Clinical Research Department, E. Merck, Darmstadt, FRG.*

Abstract

A visual search study was designed which varied the degree of automaticity of search and response decision processes by varying search set size (two or four times), mapping (consistent or variable), number of targets to be searched for (one or two targets), and number of targets to be detected (one or two targets). The observed age-related slowing of performance could be described well by one linear function. This supports the complexity hypothesis, which assumes a proportional slowing of all cognitive processes including automatic processes. Yet when the search latencies for each target were analysed separately, some inconsistencies were found that might be related to early and late selection.

Introduction

The aim of this study is to report an experiment about the relation between age on the one hand, and automatic and controlled visual search on the other.

The main objective was to test whether an age-related decrement in speed is different for automatic and controlled processes. This was accomplished by varying the degree to which the processes involved in a visual search task are either automatic or controlled. Following the brief review in Beringer *et al.* (chapter 4, this volume), one should be sceptical about assumptions of a qualitative difference. The complexity hypothesis (Cerella *et al.*, 1980) proposes a proportional age-related slowing with increasing task complexity. The automatic–controlled continuum can presumably be described simply in terms of task complexity of sheer amount of processing, rather than in terms of amount of allocated resources. There is consequently no reason why a general complexity hypothesis should fail as a description of age-related performance in automatic processes. Empirical findings by Madden and Nebes (1980), who trained young and old subjects in automatic visual search, did not show any flattening of the estimated age function with increasing automaticity. Hence, the hypothesis is that age-related speed decrement in automatic processing is qualitatively similar to that observed in controlled processing.

The first way of varying the degree of automaticity was through realizing either a consistent or a variable mapping condition. To obtain evidence whether automatic components had been established in consistent mapping, the display size was also varied (two and four items). The effect of display size is expected to be considerably larger in the variable mapping condition.

Another indication for automatic processing concerns the execution of an additional task without loss of performance. Schneider and Fisk (1982) have demonstrated that subjects can perform a dual search task without additional costs if at least one of the targets has consistent mapping and if the two targets never appear together in the same display. For this reason, a dual search condition was realized enabling the study of age-related performance with more complex visual search with automatic and controlled selection criteria depending on mapping.

Apart from this dual search—which is supposedly free of costs—another dual search task was established which is known to require nonparallel processing. Thus, Duncan (1980) found that subjects cannot simultaneously detect two targets within one display. He argued that a detected target enters the response selection stage which is not capable of processing more than one item at a time. In addition, subjects cannot unify two targets into one event. The rule used in triggering the response is therefore more complex than in dual search where only one target is present at a time. The dual task which requires the detection of two simultaneous targets will be called the dual detection condition in contrast to the dual search condition which requires detection of the one target only.

To prevent confounding task complexity with response complexity, the response was constant across all conditions. Subjects pressed a button whenever a target or, in the dual detection condition, two targets occurred. This go-no-go response was introduced for two reasons. First, it constitutes a more simple instruction (only one key to press), and second, automatic processes seem to develop faster with a go-no-go response than with a yes-no response (Van der Heijden and La Heij, 1982).

In order to facilitate the development of parallel pick-up, target and distractor stimuli belonged to different categories (letters vs. digits) in the consistent mapping condition.

Since physical similarity was expected to influence search time, context category was balanced such that half the subjects searched in a letter context and half in a digit context. The hope was to level out the effects of physical similarity and thus extend the validity of the results.

Variable mapping was expected to produce slower response latencies than consistent mapping (Schneider and Shiffrin, 1977). Dual search was expected to be in the range of single search with display size four (Schneider and Fisk, 1982) and to be faster than dual detection (Duncan, 1980).

According to the results of the studies reviewed by Beringer *et al.* (this volume), more complex conditions show larger absolute age effects, but with essentially the same slope of the age function, which relates the reaction time of old and young subjects to each other. The comparison between variable mapping and between both types of dual task will reveal to what extent automatic processes may have an age function with a different slope.

Method

Apparatus and stimuli

A DEC PDP 11/23 computer was used to present stimuli on a Hewlett-Packard Model 1332 A x-y monitor and to record response latencies. Subjects sat in a dimly lit and noise attenuated room. They responded by pushing a morse key type of button. Their head rested on a chin-rest.

The stimulus set consisted of the six upper case letters A, C, F, H, Q, and R and the six digits 1, 4, 5, 6, 7, and 8 (Figure 1). This stimulus set was selected as the best solution with regard to homogeneity of physical similarities between the various combinations of target and distractor sets. Similarity scores were taken from a study by Mohr (1984).

A single stimulus had a vertical size of 12 mm and a horizontal size of 8 mm, resulting in a vertical visual angle of 0.48°. In each trial four stimuli were displayed in each corner of a virtual square on a dark background. The visual angle of the diagonal of the virtual square (including the effective height of the stimuli) was 5.63°.

Design

On each trial a cue was presented which defined the target. Display size was varied by instructing the subjects to search only one diagonal of the virtual

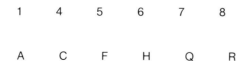

Figure 1. Set of 12 stimuli used in the experiment as targets and distractors.

square instead of searching all four positions. This method produces results that are comparable to those obtained when varying the number of actually displayed stimuli (Shiffrin and Schneider, 1977, Experiment 4a) and has the advantage of a constant complexity of the display.

The distractor set did not change during the entire experiment for each subject. One-half of the subjects searched among digits and one-half among letters. Altogether there were six different conditions. Figure 2 shows examples of a cue which defined the target and of a search display of a positive trial for each condition. To illustrate the various search sets, diagonals are included in

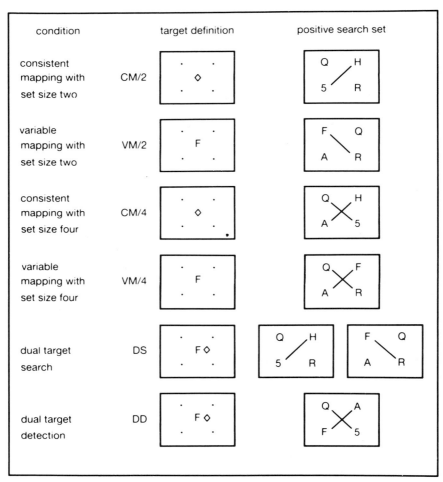

Figure 2. Examples of a target definition and a positive search set for all six conditions.

the figure; these were not displayed in the real experiment. All conditions were run in separate blocks.

In conditions one (CM/2) and two (VM/2), the search set size was two, i.e., subjects searched only one of two diagonals. In a consistent mapping condition (CM), subjects searched for a digit among letter distractors, or vice versa. In a variable mapping condition (VM), the task was to search for the target, displayed in the cue, among distractors that belonged to the same category as the target (see Figure 2); a new target was defined for each trial. For each subject consistent and variable mapping were on opposite diagonals.

Conditions three (CM/4) and four (VM/4) were identical to conditions one (CM/2) and two (VM/2) with the exception that subjects were instructed to search all four positions, i.e., both diagonals.

Condition five was a dual search (DS) condition. Subjects searched simultaneously for a consistent target on one diagonal and for a variable target on the other. Consistent and variable target search remained on the same respective diagonal as in conditions one (CM/2) and two (VM/2). Although subjects searched for two targets, only one target could appear in each display. Thus, there were two types of positive outcomes: presence of a consistent target or of a variable target.

In condition six, the targets were defined as in condition five, but they could both be present in the same display. Subjects were verbally instructed to respond only if both targets were present, so that dual detection (DD) was required. Consistent and variable target search remained on separate diagonals as in conditions one (CM/2) and two (VM/2). Negative trials always contained one target.

This set of conditions provides the possibility to compare the characteristics of subsets of treatments. Conditions CM/2 and VM/2 differ from conditions CM/4 and VM/4 in display size (two vs. four); the difference between conditions CM/4, VM/4, and DS is the number of selection criteria, other things being equal. The main difference between conditions DS and DD is the number of targets to be detected.

To avoid interference between the various conditions and to abbreviate the time taken by an experimental session, a subset of the six conditions was varied within subjects. The total sample of 30 young and 30 old subjects was split into three groups of 10 subjects each. Conditions CM/2 and VM/2 were carried out by all groups. Group one then continued with conditions CM/4 and VM/4, group two with condition DS, and group three with condition DD.

All subjects participated in two sessions. All groups started by performing conditions CM/2 and VM/2, the order of which was balanced between subjects, and each subject began with the alternative condition in the second session. In this way, CM/2 and VM/2 assumed the role of baseline conditions. After performing CM/2 and VM/2, subjects of each group ran their remaining condition(s). In group one, the order of condition CM/4 and VM/4 was also balanced between subjects and alternated in the second session. From each group of 10 subjects, five searched among digit and five among letter distractors. Sex was balanced within each group and within each age group. One-half of the subjects searched on the 45° diagonal for the consistent target and on the 135° diagonal for the variable target; this was reversed for the other half. Within each context subgroup these factors were only approximately balanced (3.2) because a cell contained only five subjects.

Subjects

Thirty young and 30 old subjects participated on a voluntary basis. To ensure maximum similarity of education background, occupation, and motivation for participation, subjects were recruited among employees of the same industrial organization, with the exception of three old subjects who worked elsewhere.

Before the experiment, subjects were screened in the laboratory of the organization. Only right-handed subjects were selected with normal or corrected vision and with no colour blindness. The mean age was 26 years for young and 57 years for old subjects. Subjects were paid for participation in the screening and in the experiment. Three old subjects were replaced after the first experimental session because they made too many errors ($> 20\%$).

Procedure

Depending on group membership, one session lasted 45–55 minutes. The first session started with 96 practice trials which were of the same type as the first condition (CM/2 or VM/2). After these practice trials, the first condition with 96 experimental trials was run. All remaining conditions consisted of 24 practice trials followed by 96 experimental trials. In the second session, the first condition was again practised with 48 trials, followed by 96 experimental trials. Subjects were allowed a five minute rest after the first two conditions.

Each target stimulus appeared with equal frequency in all four positions. Each distractor stimulus appeared equally often, while position and target-distractor combination were randomized. Probability of the target was 0.5 in all conditions.

A trial started with the cue defining the target (see Figure 3). In consistent mapping, a diamond was displayed in the centre of the display as a cue instructing the subjects to search for any of the six consistent targets. In the variable mapping condition, the target itself was displayed in the centre of the display as a cue defining the target in the next trial. In conditions DS and DD, the cue was a combination of both types: The variable target was displayed in the centre of the display, while a diamond was added to the right of the centre

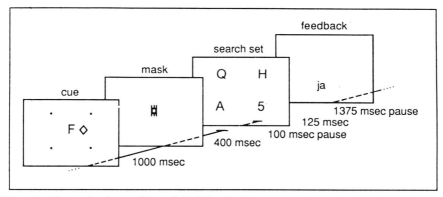

Figure 3. Example of a positive trial of the dual search condition. The letter 'F' and all of the six digits are defined as the target. Since subjects search for any digit and the search set contains the digit '5' it is appropriate to press the key here.

to emphasize the additional search for a consistent target. In Figure 3, for example, subjects searched for any digit (diamond) and for the letter 'F' as the variable target. The target was displayed for 1 s followed by a pattern mask for 400 ms in the area where the variable target was previously displayed. The pattern mask served both as a mask and as a fixation point. After a further interval of 100 ms, the search set was presented for 125 ms to avoid saccadic eye movements during actual display.

Subjects responded by pressing a button with their right index finger. Measurement of search time was started at the onset of the search set. Maximum reaction time was 1.5 s, after which a feedback signal was presented at the bottom of the screen informing the subjects whether a button press was the correct response (JA) or whether no response was required (NEIN). The feedback was displayed for 600 ms followed by an interval of 600 ms. The next trial then started automatically.

Results and Discussion

Since overall error proportions exceeded 10% for at least some of the subjects, accuracy of performance was included in the data analysis. To avoid problems of response bias and of assumptions about signal-to-noise distributions, the parameter A' (Craig, 1979) was used as an estimator of accuracy. In contrast to d', A' is a nonparametric measure averaging the upper- and lower-bound areas defined by a given point on the ROC. Although A' has a considerable measurement error, and is therefore conservative (Williams, 1980), it is supposed to be the best nonparametric alternative to d' (Craig, 1979). Mean RT and A' for each group and condition are presented in Figure 4.

Analyses of variance were carried out on both single dependent variables,

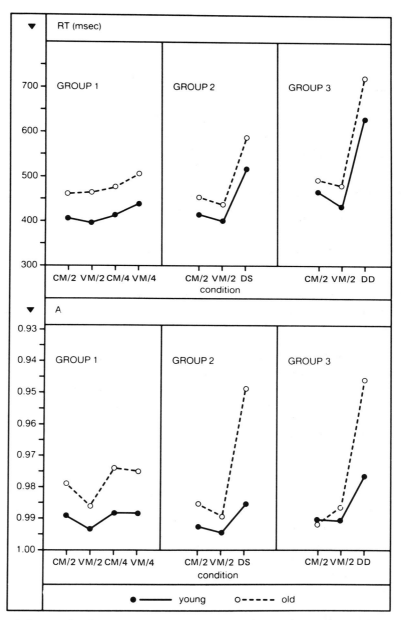

Figure 4. Interaction between age and condition CM/2, VM/2. CM/4, VM/4, DS and DD for each of the experimental groups with reaction time (RT) and A′ as the dependent variable.

and a multivariate analysis of variance was carried out with RT and A', with A' transformed by an arcsine function. The pattern of significant effects on single RT was similar to the pattern of multivariate effects on RT. Hence, single RT significances will generally be used. A' will not be considered separately, because it usually covaried with RT, which suggests the absence of a speed–accuracy trade-off (see Figure 4).

The main effects of age, session, and condition were significant in all groups, except for age in the third group. In group one, the interaction between the effects of display size was smaller for consistent targets, indicating that some degree of automaticity had developed.

In order to identify age-related decrements in performance, the interaction between the effects of age and condition is usually considered. Virtually no interaction was obtained in group one, but age differences increased in the dual task (DS and DD) relative to the baseline conditions in groups two and three. In group two, the interaction between single (CM/2 and VM/2) and dual (DS) tasks was significant ($P < .001$). in group three, the interaction effect was only marginally significant in the multivariable analysis of variance ($P < . 1.$).

This pattern of results does not necessarily indicate a specific age-related decrement in dual task processing. As argued earlier, one should consider the proportional relations between age differences and different levels of task complexity in order to decide whether specific deficits are involved. Estimates of age function by considering reaction times of the conditions CM/2, VM/2, CM/4, VM/4, DS, and DD can provide information about the extent to which the proportion of the reaction time of young and old subjects remains constant as postulated by the complexity hypothesis. The age function was estimated by means of the mean RTs of each condition and context (letter, digit) subgroup, so that 12 data points were available. Figure 5 shows the resulting age function, which fits the data quite well ($r = 0.94$). The slope value of 1.20 is the range of values obtained in other experiments.

The age function was also estimated with corrected means on the basis of baseline performance (CM/2 and VM/2). For each subject the mean RT of both baseline conditions was subtracted from that of the remaining conditions. In this way individual and group differences are largely eliminated, and the residual variance is mainly due to additional task complexity. Figure 6 shows the corrected data points together with the age function. With the remaining eight points the fit is somewhat better ($r = 0.99$) than with the uncorrected values. The slope of 1.28 is slightly more than that obtained by means of the uncorrected values but comes close to an average of 1.3 reported in Cerella *et al.* (1980).

The fact that age-related performance can be well described by a single age function favours, of course, the notion of a general slowing of all processes involved in visual search. The question is, however, whether a more detailed analysis of the data will provide additional evidence for a unique slowing

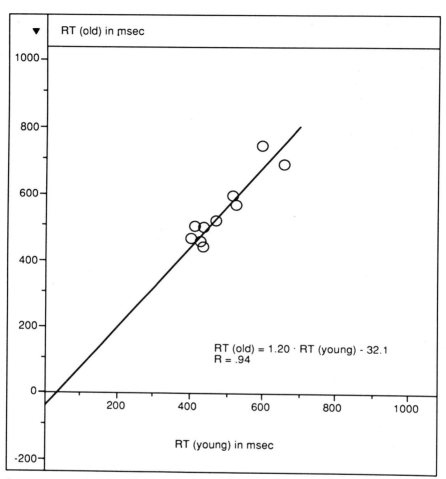

2 circles coincidental

Figure 5. Estimated age function and mean reaction times (RT) of old and young subjects for the six experimental conditions and each context group separately.

factor. Thus, search latencies of the baseline conditions CM/2 and VM/2 were analysed for each target separately. An analysis of variance was carried out with group and age as between-subject factors and mapping (consistent vs. variable) and target identity as within-subject factors. Target identity was analysed as a within-subject factor, although the repeated measurement was in fact crossed between mapping and target category according to context group.

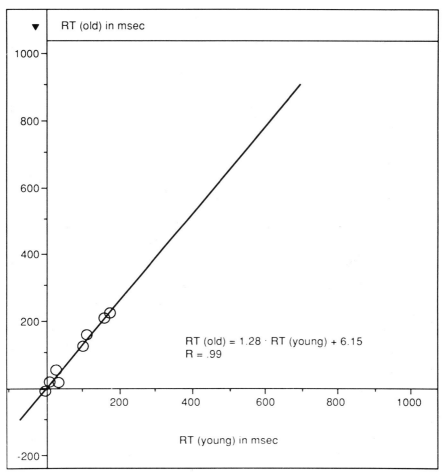

Figure 6. Estimated age function and corrected mean reaction times (RT) of old and young subjects for CM/4, VM/4, DS, and DD. Reaction times are corrected by subtracting the mean of the baseline conditions CM/2 and VM/2 of the first session.

For example, a consistent digit target belonged to the letter context group, whereas a consistent letter belonged to the digit context group. The mean reaction times are shown in Figure 7. Each data point is based on 240 observations for each age, mapping and target combination. The main effect of target identity ($P < .001$) and the interaction between the effects of target identity, mapping, and age ($P < .001$) were highly significant. These data cannot be explained by one linear age function.

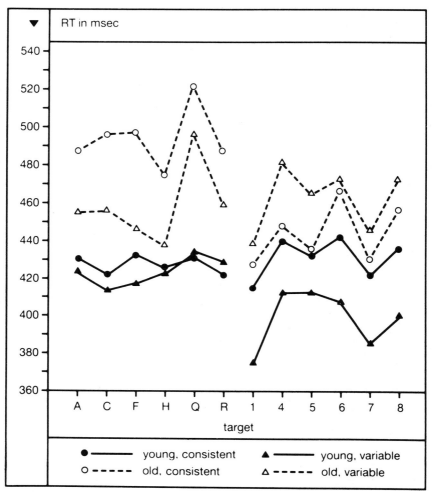

Figure 7. Reaction times (RT) of young and old subjects for each target and mapping condition in the baseline conditions CM/2 and VM/2.

Conclusions

Our finding that the reaction times of all conditions fit one function suggests a common age-related slowing factor for both automatic and controlled processes in search and response selection. This is in line with the complexity hypothesis (Cerella *et al.*, 1980) and with the brief description of attention in Beringer *et al.* (chapter 4, this volume).

Our experiment at the same time demonstrates, however, that the complexity hypothesis does not suffice to describe all age-related differences in information processing. Mean latencies for each target (see Figure 7) cannot be described by one linear age function. These inconsistencies must be discussed in terms of their impact on the notion of a general age-related slowing factor.

The effect of target identity is most likely due to differences in physical similarity of the items. Especially the letter 'Q' was difficult to detect for old but not for young subjects, possible because of its small discriminating diagonal. Following the argumentation in Beringer *et al.* (chapter 4, this volume), age-related differences arising from physical similarity effects are not expected to be consistent with the notion of a general slowing factor. If information pick-up of old subjects is more noisy, thus reducing the quality of the information that is available for further processing, more than speed factors are contributing to the effect of age.

In addition to physical similarity, search latencies are also affected by category membership of the target. For old subjects variably mapped letter targets were searched faster than consistently mapped letter targets, whereas the opposite is true for digit targets.

Schneider and Shiffrin (1977, Experiment 2b) did not obtain the usual advantage of consistent mapping, either, when display size was two and memory size one. The unexpected ranking of the mapping conditions might be due to the fact that mapping, as realized in this experiment, is confounded with target set size. In the case of consistent mapping six potential targets could appear during one trial, whereas in variable mapping only one target was defined. At display size two, the advantage of smaller target set size seems to level out the disadvantage of variable mapping. When display size increases, however, the disadvantage of variable mapping outweighs the advantage of display size.

In contrast to old subjects, young subjects worked with letter targets almost independently of the mapping condition, whereas variably mapped digit targets were search much faster than consistently mapped digit targets.

There is no conclusive explanation why age-related performance varies between and within target categories. It at least indicates that early (physical similarity) and late (semantic category) selection components are contributing to the search latencies at the same time.

Acknowledgements

The authors highly appreciate the support of Marion Eisele, Patricia Gropp, and Sabine Rinck for preparing and performing the experiment.

References

Cerella J, Poon LW and Williams DM (1980) Age and the complexity hypothesis. In: Poon LW (ed.) *Aging in the 1980s: Psychological Issues.* Washington D.C.: American Psychological Association.

Craig A (1979) Nonparametric measures of sensory efficiency for sustained monitoring tasks. *Hum. Factors* **21**, 67–79.

Duncan J (1980) The locus of interference in the perception of simultaneous stimuli. *Psychol. Rev.* **87**, 272–300.

Madden DJ and Nebes D (1980) Aging and the development of automaticity in visual search. *Dev. Psychol.* **16** 377–84.

Mohr W (1984) *Visuelle Wahrnehmung und Zeichenfunktion: Untersuchungen zur Grundlage des Kategorieneffekts bei der Wahrnehmung von Buchstaben und Ziffern.* Regensburg: Roderer.

Schneider W and Fisk AD (1982) Concurrent automatic and controlled visual search: can processing occur without resource cost? *J. Exp. Psychol.: Learning, Memory, and Cognition* **8**, 261–78.

Schneider W and Shiffrin RM (1977) Controlled and automatic human processing: I. Detection, search, and attention *Psychol. Rev.* **84**, 1–66.

Shiffrin RM and Schneider W (1977) Controlled and automatic human processing: II. Perceptual learning, automatic attending, and a general theory. *Psychol. Rev.* **84**, 127–90.

Van der Heijden AHC and La Heij W (1982) The array size function in simple visual search tasks: A comparison between 'go-no go' and 'yes-no' tasks under conditions of high and low target-noise similarity. *Psychol. Res.* **44**, 355–68.

Williams MV (1980) Receiver operating characteristics: The effect of distribution on between-group comparisons. In: Poon LW (ed.) *Aging in the 1980s: Psychological Issues.* Washington D.C.: American Psychological Association.

Psychopharmacology and Reaction Time
Edited by I. Hindmarch, B. Aufdembrinke and H. Ott
©1988 John Wiley & Sons Ltd.

6

Some Boundary Conditions of Choice Reaction Performance

Donald Laming

*Department of Experimental Psychology, University of Cambridge,
Cambridge, UK*

Abstract

Most studies of the effects of drugs on reaction time have been analysed using Sternberg's additive—factor method. This method depends on a) an analytic model based on an idea—decomposition into canonical components—of very wide applicability in physical science; and b) a specific psychological interpretation—the canonical components are taken to be successive stages in the translation from stimulus to response.

Here I apply the *same* analytic model to the *same* generic class of experiments, but coupled with a *different* psychological interpretation, in which the canonical components are taken to be *boundary conditions* of some presently unknown choice reaction process. In this way the effects of trial-to-trial feedback following an error can be modelled with only very simple and unexceptionable assumptions about the underlying process. The effects of this experimental variable admit simple quantitative models which may, for that reason, provide useful indicators of the effects of drugs on reaction time.

Introduction

Choice reaction (CR) performance fluctuates from trial to trial in a manner which is related to preceding events, notably stimuli, errors, and latencies. In this chapter, I show how these naturally occurring perturbations in CR performance may be analysed, and I suggest that they might be used to monitor the effects of drugs and other stressors.

Of necessity, *preceding* events influence *present* performance via certain internal parameters of the CR process. Such internal parameters might be

65

likened to the boundary conditions imposed on the solution of a partial differential equation. Just as the motion of water through a pipe is constrained by the geometry of the channel in which it flows, so CR performance depends on the momentary values of its internal parameters. Envisage that these momentary values are adjusted from trial to trial in the light of feedback from the experimental task; sequential fluctuations are thereby generated. To illustrate this, I shall set out my present conjectures what some of these internal parameters are, together with the principal evidence (concerning the after-effects of an error) on which my conjectures are based.

Linear Analysis of Reaction Time Data

Suppose that the observed reaction time (RT) is a smooth function of several variables x_a, x_b, x_c, ...;

$$\mathrm{RT} = T(x_a,\ x_b,\ x_c,\ ...) \tag{1}$$

I do not wish to identify the variables at this point, though I have in mind such factors as stimulus probability, foreperiod, and accuracy, and I shall treat the variables as continuous. Now induce small perturbations δx_a, δx_b, δx_c, ... in these variables about equilibrium values x_a', x_b', x_c', ... Then

$$\mathrm{RT} = T(x_a',\ x_b',\ x_c',\ ...) +$$
$$+ \frac{\delta T}{\delta x_a}\delta x_a + \frac{\delta T}{\delta x_b}\delta x_b + \frac{\delta T}{\delta x_c}\delta x_c + ... \tag{2}$$

The perturbation δx_a might be induced, for example, by the preceding stimulus – on trial n this would be S_{n-1}. Then, still without identifying the variable x_a,

$$\delta_a RT = \frac{\delta T}{\delta x_a}\delta x_a \tag{3}$$

measures the effect of S_{n-1} on RT_n. By adding to Eq. 2 as many terms as one thinks fit, each term representing some preceding event in the experiment, the possible effects of these preceding events on present performance can be analysed. This method can be applied to responses as well as latencies. The details have been set out by Laming (1968).

To relate this procedure for the analysis of sequential fluctuations to more familiar methods, I remark that Eqs. 2 and 3 are *formally* the same as the equations recommended by Sternberg (1969) with his additive factors method. And that method is now widely used for the analysis of RT data, especially on the effects of drugs (e.g., Frowien, 1981; Logsdon *et al.*, 1984). Sternberg's method involves two independent elements:

1. An analytic model (Eq. 2) based on an idea—decomposition into canonical components—of very wide applicability in physical science
2. A specific psychological interpretation: the canonical components are taken to be successive independent stages in the translation from stimulus into response

I have used the *same* analytic model. But its validity is in no way dependent on its psychological interpretation. To show this is so, I will suggest an alternative.

Many processes in physical science are specified by differential equations that describe *local* behaviour. A particularly pertinent example is Brownian motion which, in one dimension, satisfies the equation

$$\frac{1}{2} \sigma^2 \frac{\delta^2 f}{\delta x^2} - \mu \frac{\delta f}{\delta x} = \frac{\delta f}{\delta t} \tag{4}$$

This example is pertinent because Eq. 4 describes the local behaviour of a normally distributed random walk, and this stochastic process has been studied as a candidate model for choice reaction time (CRT) by several investigators (Stone, 1960; Fitts, 1966; Laming, 1968; Link, 1975; Green *et al.*, 1983; Green and von Gierke, 1984).

The random walk (Eq. 4) evolves in two dimensions—time and space. It is uniform in time, but random in the spatial dimension, and evolves in this way until it reaches one of two absorbing boundaries. Suppose these boundaries are set at $x = a$ and $x = b$. Because the walk is random in the spatial dimension, the time taken to reach one of these boundaries is also a random variable, and is commonly identified with the decision component of CRT. The distribution of that decision component depends on a and b, which are—exactly—boundary conditions of the differential equation.

I envisage that the location of these boundaries—the values a and b—might be adjusted from trial to trial, especially after an error. I envisage that there might be other boundary conditions as well—for example, the epoch at which the decision process begins—which are adjusted in like manner. So what follows is a summary of my present conjectures about some of the boundary conditions within which CRs evolve based upon analyses of trial-to-trial fluctuations in my own experiments. These fluctuations occur naturally and are related to preceding events—stimuli, errors, latencies—in the experiment. Those preceding events communicate their effects to present performance through certain, presently unknown, internal parameters of the CR process. My objective is to build up a picture of that process by identifying its internal parameters. It may be that this picture will permit certain significant classes of CR models to be excluded from further consideration.

Figure 1 summarizes my present conjectures in diagrammatic form. It will guide the reader through the remainder of this chapter. I emphasize *present*

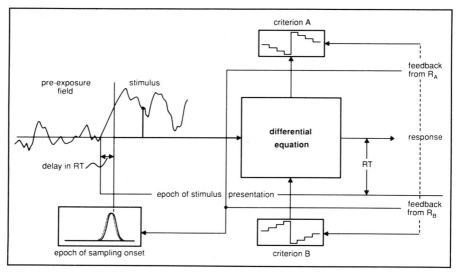

Figure 1. A diagrammatic summary of some of the mechanisms and their interactions which are conjectured to generate the sequential phenomena observed in choice reaction experiments.

conjectures because there are several different species of fluctuation in CR performance and my views might yet change about their classification into phylogenetic families. I also emphasize that these conjectures are based solely on analyses of my own data because, with the partial exception of two papers by Green *et al.* (1983) and Green and von Gierke (1984), there are no other comparable analyses to hand.

The Experiments

Full details of the experiments have been published elsewhere (Laming, 1968). Here I give only a brief description.

The stimuli were two vertical white stripes 0.50 in. wide and 4.00 in. (S_A) and 2.83 in. (S_B) high. These stripes were mounted on black cards and exposed in a multiple Dodge tachistoscope about 3 m in front of the subject's eyes. The stimulus remained available to the subject's inspection until he responded by pressing one of two keys with one or the other forefinger. Typically, an experiment involved 24 subjects who each contributed five blocks of 200 trials for analysis following as short period of practice. The employment of such a large number of subjects permits a simple nonparametric (binomial) test of each different sequential statistic against between-subject variation.

At this point caution is called for. Some of the boundary conditions of the CR process are implicit in the design of the experiment—for example, in the choice of the foreperiod (cf. Green *et al.*, 1983). So not all of the results which are statistically significant in my data will generalize to other experiments.

The After-effects of an Error

I envisage that the local evolution of an individual CR decision process will ultimately admit description by a partial differential equation; but I do not wish, yet, to say what I think that equation will turn out to be. I have previously looked on Eq. 4 as a plausible candidate. But I do not now think that random walk models are appropriate; and the survey which follows will be conducted without any specific assumption about the nature of the CR process. The box in Figure 1 labelled *Differential equation*, which generates the *Response* after the measured *RT*, is accordingly left empty.

The number of response criteria

I begin, however, by demonstrating one fundamental property which must be incorporated in that box. Figure 2 shows the mean RTs and proportions of errors (PEs), separately for each of the stimuli, from an experiment (Laming, 1968, Experiment 2) in which the proportions of each stimulus were varied, as shown, from one block of trials to another. It is clear that mean RT depends on the stimulus in such a way that the more frequent stimulus elicits the fast response. Since the identity of the stimulus is not known to the subject in advance, the period for which the stimulus is inspected *cannot be prede-termined*. A two-choice reaction is therefore a *sequential* process with *two* response criteria C_A and C_B. It continues until one of these criteria is satisfied. so the differential equation in Figure 1 involves time as one of its variables; and the two criteria are explicitly represented as two boundary conditions (*Criterion* A and *Criterion* B) of the CR process.

Performance following an error

I next examine what happens after the subject has made an error. Figure 3 shows the PEs and the variation in mean RT on trials immediately following an error in this same experiment and in two others similar to it (Laming, 1968, Experiments 1, 2, and 3). If e is the number of the trial on which the error occurs, then the subject takes longer to respond on trials $(e + 1)$, $(e + 2)$, and $(e + 3)$, and is less likely than usual to make a further error. The subject takes greater care. This effect is observed for *both* responses, but is more pro-nounced for the *response* uttered in error. The increment in RT is greater if the alternate stimulus is presented so that the response uttered in error is required a second time; and there is a corresponding difference in the depression of the PE (Laming, 1979a). So when response R_i has been uttered in error, there must be some adjustment to its criterion C_i, but not necessarily to the other criterion, making it less likely that R_i will be uttered in error again. Consequently, R_i takes longer if it is required on the succeeding trial. I go on to explore the immediate implications of this idea.

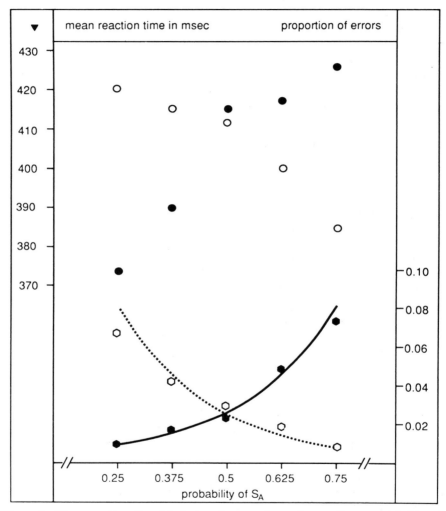

Figure 2. Mean reaction time (circles) and proportions of erros (hexagons) in Experiment 2 from Laming (1968). Open symbols relate to Stimulus A, filled symbols to Stimulus B. The *curves* fitted to the proportions of errors are calculated according to Eqs. 6. (From Laming 1969. Copyright 1969 Academic Press. Reproduced by permission.)

Adjustments to response criteria

Suppose that after R_i has been uttered in error, its criterion C_i is increased by an amount ΔC. Since no progressive decrease in the probabilities of error is observed in the course of the experiment, there must be some countervailing

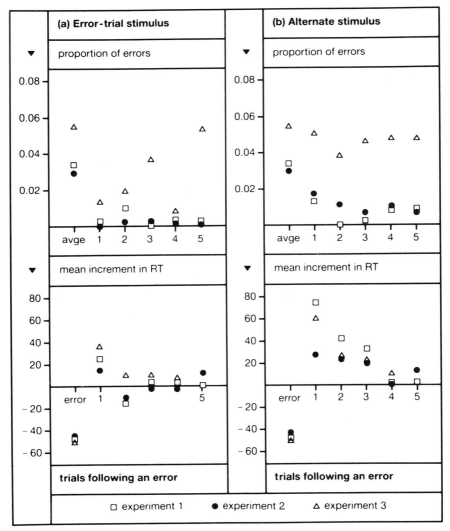

Figure 3. Proportions of errors and mean increments in reaction time on the five trials following an error in Experiments 1, 2, and 3 from Laming (1968). (From Laming 1979a. Copyright 1979 by the North-Holland Publishing Co. Reproduced by permission.)

decrease of C_i whenever R_i is correct. The size of that decrease δC must be much smaller than ΔC, because correct responses are much more frequent than errors. So the succession of responses R_i, correct responses and errors, will cause the criterion C_i to fluctuate in a dynamic equilibrium about the point where

$$(1 - \epsilon)\,\delta C = \epsilon\,\Delta C, \tag{5}$$

ϵ being the equilibrium probability of error contingent on the response. This dynamic adjustment is represented by the staircases within the boxes labelled criterion A and criterion B in Figure 1.

If the same ΔC and δC apply to both criteria, the contingent probability of error ϵ will be the same for both responses. Suppose now that S_B is presented with probability p and S_A with probability $1 - p$. Then the probability of error *contingent on the stimuli* can be shown by calculation to be (see Laming, 1968, p. 33):

$$\alpha = P(R_B|S_A) = \epsilon(p - \epsilon)/(1 - p)(1 - 2\epsilon)$$

$$\tag{6}$$

$$\beta = P(R_A|S_B) = \epsilon(1 - p - \epsilon)/p(1 - 2\epsilon).$$

Equations 6 are shown as the curves fitted to the proportions of errors in Figure 2.

It would be natural to propose a corresponding relation between stimulus probability and mean RT. But that presupposes a decision model to relate latency to accuracy, occupying the box labelled *Differential equation* in Figure 1. I prefer not to introduce any such model at this juncture.

Epoch of sampling onset

I return to Figure 3: If R_A is uttered in error, the subject knows that criterion C_A is too lax and needs to be adjusted; but there is no feedback from C_B. Yet a significant increase in RT and a complementary decrease in PE are observed on trial $(e + 1)$ for *both* responses. I conjecture that the results in Figure 3 reflect *two* distinct adjustments following an error, one to the response criteria which affects only that response uttered in error, and another adjustment which affects both responses equally.

The subject cannot judge *exactly* when the reaction stimulus will be presented. I suggest that, in these experiments with fixed intertrial intervals, he selects an epoch in advance at which he begins examining the stimulus display to decide whether it is S_A or S_B which he is looking at. If that *epoch of sampling onset* comes *after* the stimulus has been presented, the recorded RT is increased by exactly that delay. Such a delay is illustrated explicitly in Figure 1. If sampling begins *before* the stimulus is presented, the reaction process begins with the analysis of 'noise' from the pre-exposure field, analysed as though it were the reaction stimulus, and for most random processes occurring in nature this noise will increase the probability of error in roughly exponential fashion. These two effects are represented diagrammatically in Figure 4.

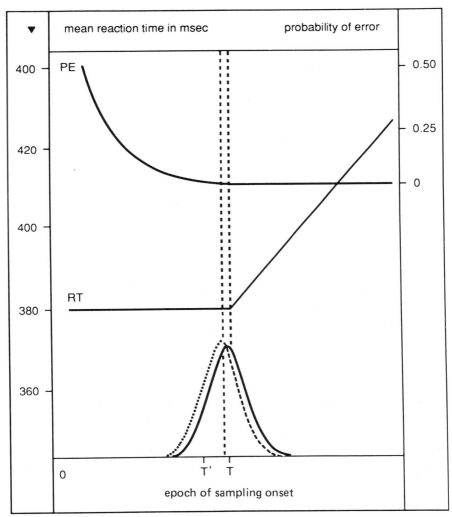

Figure 4. A diagram to illustrate the likely variation of the probability of error and of the measured reaction time as functions of the hypothetical epoch of sampling onset. The *lower part* of the figure shows two possible distributions of this epoch together with the contribution (*broken line*) of the dotted distribution to measured reaction time. (From Laming 1979b. Copyright 1979 by the North-Holland Publishing Co. Reproduced by permission.)

The epoch of sampling onset cannot, however, be selected precisely, because the subject's estimation of even a fixed intertrial interval is subject to a large error—large relative to the variability of a reaction time in these experiments (see Laming, 1968, p. 81). This error of estimation is represented by the distribution (two alternatives are shown) in the lower part of Figure 4 and also in the box labelled *epoch of sampling onset* in Figure 1. The range of sampling onsets covered by one or the other of these distributions will, on some trials, produce a real time increase in the recorded RT and, on others, an exponential increase in the probability of error.

Choice reaction performance is characterized by a compromise between these two aberrations, affecting speed and accuracy respectively, and all that the subject can do following an error is retard the distribution of epochs by some suitable amount, producing the decrease in probability of error and the real time increase in RT for *both* responses that can be seen in Figure 3.

Autocorrelation of RTs

Since the probability of error does not uniformly decrease during continued CR performance, there must, after each correct response, be a small advance of the distribution of the sampling epoch. I envisage that each epoch of sampling onset is a *random* readjustment of the value, relative to the presentation of the reaction stimulus, on the preceding trial, so that epochs selected on successive trials are positively correlated. To the extent that these epochs come after the presentation of the reaction stimulus, they make positively correlated contributions to successive reaction times. Figure 5 shows the correlations between successive RTs in five different experiments; they fit nicely (within ± 1.95 s.e.s.) to the equation

$$r_k = 0.125(0.721)^{k-1} \tag{7}$$

which is represented by the continuous curve. I attribute these autocorrelations to the presumed correlations between delays of the epoch of sampling onset on successive trials. It is interesting that Experiment 5 (see Laming, 1968, p. 64) compared five different values of fixed intertrial (response-stimulus) intervals ranging from 1 to 4096 msec. There was no difference in autocorrelation between those five chosen intervals, suggesting that the mechanism of that correlation is driven by the succession of stimulus presentations rather than by other events in real time.

Comparable analyses of changes in performance on the trial following an error and of autocorrelations of RT have been published by Green *et al.* (1983) and by Green and von Gierke (1984). These authors found much smaller autocorrelation coefficients—never greater than 0.07 and usually negligible— and no consistent increase in RT or decrease in PE on the trial following an error. In their experiments the foreperiod which separated the presentation

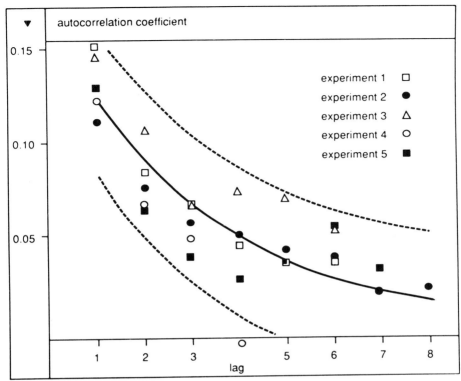

Figure 5. Median serial correlation coefficients from five experiments by Laming (1968). The *broken curves* delimit 0.95 confidence intervals about the *continuous curve* which has Eq. 7. (From Laming 1979b. Copyright by the North-Holland Publishing Co. Reproduced by permission.)

of the reaction stimulus from the warning signal varied at random with an *exponential* distribution up to a maximum of 6238 msec. This means that their subjects could have had *no knowledge whatever* of when the reaction stimulus would be presented. So it was impossible in their experiments to select a sampling epoch that bore any other than a completely random relation to the presentation of the reaction stimulus. The mechanism that I have conjectured could not have operated in those exponential foreperiod experiments. It does not follow, however, that Green's subjects did not sample the pre-exposure field. Green *et al.* reported small numbers of *anticipations* for all subjects under all conditions; that is, on some very small numbers of trials, the subjects uttered choice responses before the reaction stimulus appeared. In the visual experiment (Green and von Gierke, 1984) errors were not independent of the foreperiod; fewer errors were uttered after the shortest foreperiods.

Conclusions

The great part of this chapter has been a statement of my present conjectures about the nature and interrelations of the different sequential effects which may be discovered following an error in two-choice reaction experiments together with the principal evidence on which those conjectures are based. This evidence is drawn solely from my own experiments because, with very few exceptions, analyses of other CR experiments in comparable detail have not been published. The unrepresentative sample of evidence that I have presented here is all that exists at this present time.

My method of analysing sequential effects in CR performance bears a close relation to Sternberg's additive-factors method: it uses the same analytic model. The psychological interpretation is different, however, as also are the experimental factors which are entered as independent variables into that model. Because of the kinds of independent variables in which I am interested, I find it more helpful to make analogy with the boundary conditions which constrain the realization of some physical process characterized by a partial differential equation, and Brownian motion is an excellent and very pertinent example of the kind of analogy I have in mind.

The practical usefulness of sequential effects subsists in the fact that they may be studied, as here, without any prior model for the fundamental CR process. The very mild assumption that RT and PE are smooth (though unknown) functions of the variables of interest is sufficient. In combination with Eq. 2 this assumption supports a quantitative analysis of a wide range of effects. This commends sequential effects in general as interesting vehicles for studying the effects of drugs on reaction processes. I have found experiments with as few as 24 000 trials (in total) sufficient to demonstrate differences in RT of less than 5 msec and differences in PE of less than 0.01—differences that are statistically significant with respect to between-subject variability. So the potential indicators of pharmacological effects look to be very sensitive. Moreover, studies of the effects of drugs on these sequential effects are likely to produce some valuable feedback to the purely psychological problem of the nature of CRTs.

References

Fitts PM (1966) Cognitive aspects of information processing: III. set for speed versus accuracy. *J. Exp. Psychol.* **71**, 849–57.

Frowein HW (1981) Selective effects of barbiturate and amphetamine on information processing and response execution *Acta Psychol.* **47**, 105–15.

Green DM von Gierke SM (1984) Visual and auditory choice reaction times. *Acta Psychol.* **55**, 231–47.

Green DM, Smith AF von Gierke SM (1983). Choice reaction time with a random foreperiod. *Percept. Psychophysics* **34**, 195–208.

Laming DRJ (1969) *Information Theory of Choice-Reaction Times.* London: Academic Press.

Laming DRJ (1969) Subjective probability in choice-reaction experiments *J. Math. Psychol.* **6**, 81–120.

Laming DRJ (1979a) Choice reaction performance following an error. *Acta Psychol.* **43**, 199–224.

Laming DRJ (1979b.) Autocorrelation of choice-reaction times. *Acta Psychol.*, **43**, 381–412.

Link SW (1975) The relative judgment theory of two choice response time. *J. Math. Psychol.* **12**, 114–35.

Logsdon R, Hochhaus L, Williams HL, Rundell OH and Maxwell D. (1984) Secobarbital and perceptual processing. *Acta Psychol.* **55**, 179–93.

Sternberg S (1969) The discovery of processing stages: Extensions of Donder's method. In: Koster WG (ed.) *Attention and Performance II.* Amsterdam: North-Holland. pp. 276–315

Stone M (1960) Models for choice-reaction time. *Psychometrika* **25**, 51–60.

Psychopharmacology and Reaction Time
Edited by I. Hindmarch, B. Aufdembrinke and H. Ott
© 1988 John Wiley & Sons Ltd.

7

The Faster the Better? Some Comments on the Use of Information Processing Rate as an Index of Change and Individual Differences in Performance

P. M. A. Rabbitt

Age and Cognitive Performance Research Centre, University of Manchester, Manchester, UK

Abstract

Information processing speed has been treated as a cardinal index of changes in efficiency of performance under stress or drugs, and more recently as a central explanatory variable in interpretations of the effects of ageing and of individual differences in intelligence. Some logical and methodological difficulties with use of simple measures of information processing rate for these purposes are illustrated by seven experiments evaluating the effects of age, alcohol and individual differences in intelligence on performance of tests of reaction time and recognition memory efficiency.

Introduction

Current models in cognitive psychology must remain crude approximations until they can overcome two related limitations: they are models of hypothetical 'steady state' systems which do not describe change, and they are models of hypothetical standard systems which do not describe individual differences. In actual fact, the human cognitive system is radically changed by practice and the acquisition of new data. As the brain matures through childhood, decays in senescence, or is perturbed by damage, illness, or drugs, tasks are not merely performed with more or less efficiency, but in radically different ways. It is also obviously incorrect to assume that all cognitive systems are identical and that individual differences contribute much less variance than differences in experimental conditions. The most important challenge to cognitive psychology is to produce adequate models of cognitive change and individual differences (Rabbitt, 1981).

A simple way to adapt current steady state models to explain change and individual différences is to find a single index, common to most models, in terms of which individual differences and changes in performance can be interpreted. Since Hick's (1952) and Hyman's (1953) classic experiments, the rate of information processing has been a standard index derivable from most experimental paradigms and incorporated in most models of cognitive processes. It has become fashionable to use this as a critical dimension for individual differences. For example, Band and Dearie (1982), Eysenck (1985), Jensen (1985), Vernon (1983) and others have noted correlations between individual differences in IQ test scores and in speed of choice reaction time (CRT) or latency of perceptual discrimination in simple tasks. Some of these authors suggest that individual differences of CRT or inspection time may directly reflect characteristic differences in the efficiency of basic units in the CNS, such as speed of synaptic conduction or differences in neural signal-to-noise ratios (Eysenck, 1985; Hendricksen, 1982). It is congenial for those who wish to argue that differences in IQ test scores reflect inheritable biological differences to explain individual differences in problem solving ability in such terms (Jensen, 1985).

In similar vein, Salthouse (1985) suggests that a reduction of information processing speed is the most marked concomitant of old age, and he has based a general theory of cognitive ageing on this single dimension of observable change.

This chapter reviews experiments which test the limits to which this attractively simple 'single factor' hypothesis can be taken. The aim is not to offer new models for IQ, for cognitive changes in age, or even for the effect of alcohol on psychomotor performance, but rather to reveal the methodological and theoretical assumptions between which we must choose in order to adapt our present, unsatisfactory, cognitive models to account for changes within, and differences between, the systems which they represent.

Speed, Errors, Strategy and Task Demands

Changes of the information processing rate can manifest themselves either as changes of response speed or of accuracy. Which index changes will depend both on the volunteer's interpretation of experimental instructions and on the degrees of freedom which the experiment allows. Table 1 presents data from two experiments carried out by Maylor and Rabbitt (in preparation) on the same 36 volunteers aged 19–34 years who took either 0 ml, 0.33 ml, or 1.0 ml alcohol per kg body weight on different days in counterbalanced order. During these three sessions, they experienced an average of 250 trials on an easy

Table 1. Mean latencies of correct decisions, standard deviations for decision latencies, and error rates for items in a continuous, serial CRT task and in a visual search task (letter cancellation task) made by volunteers after ingesting 0 ml, 0.33 ml. and 1.0 ml alcohol per kg body weight

	Dosage of alcohol (ml/kg body weight)		
Serial choice reaction task	0 ml	0.33 ml	1.0 ml
Mean correct RT (msec)	505.8	499.3	544.0
sd correct RT	128.8	123.7	153.2
Mean error RT (msec)	468.5	469.8	521.3
sd error RT	91.0	99.2	122.7
% errors	5.1	4.1	5.1
Visual search task			
Total items scanned	5685.8	5425.3	5786.0
% false alarms	0.02	0.03	0.03
% target misses	21.4	19.5	25.9

four-choice serial self-paced CRT task. They also carried out a visual search task: this consisted in scanning printed sheets of letters as fast as possible for the target numerals 1 and 0 which occurred with a frequency of 2% among random sequences of distractor symbols (all possible upper and lower case letters including 1 and O). Table 1 shows means, standard deviations, and error rates for the CRT task, and total numbers of items scanned during five 2-minute runs, percentages of targets missed (omissions), percentages of false positives in the visual search task.

We see that in the serial CRT task alcohol reduced speed but not accuracy, while in the visual search task scanning rate was unaffected, but target omissions increased. These two paradigms have classically been discussed as logically identical. Recall that the title of Neisser's 1963 paper on visual search was *Decision time without reaction time*. But Hick (1952) had already pointed out that response speed and errors can be traded off against each other or 'equivocated' to maintain constancy of information transmission rate across different experimental conditions. To some extent, within any particular task, a person can freely choose any given trade-off or equivocation between speed and errors. But the two paradigms restrict the freedom of choice in different ways. In the serial CRT paradigm, volunteers had to make some response to each signal before the next appeared. We also know that in tasks of this type, volunteers recognize nearly all the errors that they make. Visual search paradigms do not compel volunteers to categorize every symbol on a display, and we know that most omissions go undetected (Rabbitt and Vyas, 1977).

Since volunteers get little or no feedback from most of their errors, perhaps the best that they can do is to try to maintain constant speed. Thus, although the effects of alcohol on performance can be described as a slowing of the information processing rate, the way in which this change appears can be determined by the free choice of the volunteers on whom the experiment is run, by their idiosyncratic preconceptions or interpretations of the experimental instructions and, most importantly, by the precise feedback which the task allows.

The Unit Log Hypothesis

The simplest model relating slowing of information transmission to hypothetical CNS events was made explicit by Birren *et al.* (1979). Every decision, such as that involved in identifying a signal and selecting a response, may be supposed to successively involve some finite number (N) of unitary and serial operations in the CNS. Conditions such as old age, stupidity, or ingestion of alcohol may add a constant lag (L msec) to the time taken for each of the N operations. Thus, the age of alcohol lag in any task will be the product of the number of unitary operations and the size of the unit lag ($N \cdot L$). It follows that performance of more complex tasks, which arguably require a larger N, will be proportionately more slowed than simple tasks with fewer operations. Birren *et al.* (1979) review very many studies in which older and younger people were compared on simple and more complex reaction time (RT) tasks. In all cases the expected interaction between age and task complexity appeared, i.e., old people were relatively slower on the more complex versions of the tasks. A similar logic underlies Jensen's (1985) discussion of experiments by Vernon in which volunteers with high and low IQ test scores were given a series of easy and more difficult CRT tasks. Jensen argues that differences between high and low IQ groups increase with task difficulty, though this is not clearly apparent from the data he presents.

This attractively simple picture unfortunately should not be taken at face value. We have discussed the difficulty of evaluating data from tasks in which volunteers have different possibilities of trading off speed against accuracy. Another problem is that in Vernon's studies, and in all the experiments discussed by Birren, volunteers received very little practice. Thus, older people or people with low IQs may have been particularly handicapped in the more complex versions of the tasks because they required relatively more practice to master them. Gilchrist and Rabbitt (unpublished) matched two groups of elderly (70–78 years) and young (20–24 years) volunteers on the Mill Hill vocabulary test scores and gave them each 10 days of practice on two-choice, four-choice, and eight-choice versions of a serial self-paced CRT task. Over the first five days of practice, age and task complexity interacted to determine mean RT, just as Birren *et al.* (1979) concluded. But pooled means for the last

Table 2. Mean latencies (msec) in a lexical decision task and in difficult and in easy categorization tasks by volunteers after ingesting 0 ml or 1 ml alcohol per kg body weight

	Alcohol intake		
Lexical decision task	0 ml/kg	1 ml/kg	diff.
Decision times for high freq. words	595	660	65
Decision times for medium freq. words	680	755	75
Decision times for low freq. words	755	805	50
Categorization tasks			
Decision times for semantic cat.	722	750	23
Decision times for surface cat.	664	721	56

two days of practice showed no such interaction, Rather, mean RTs for the older group showed a constant lag across all conditions.

Table 2 presents CRTs from two levels of difficulty of a lexical decision task and from a semantic and a surface categorization task (Kingstone *et al.*, in preparation) under 0 ml or 1.0 ml alcohol per kg body weight. In both comparisons, alcohol produced a similar lag in CRT for both easy and difficult conditions. The interactions between decision difficulty and alcohol effects predicted by the unit lag hypotheses did not occur.

It seems that the unit lag hypothesis is too simplistic to take into consideration the actual demands for adaptive control which even apparently trivial tasks make on the human cognitive system.

More Complex Interpretations of Efficiency Changes

Hypotheses directly relating differences in mean CRT to efficiency of individual CNS units consider the human information processing system as an entirely passive device in which a linear series of discrete, nonoverlapping, and successive transactions invariably occur in an unmodifiable order. All these premises now seem dubious, both on theoretical (Townsend and Ashby, 1983) and empirical (Rabbit 1980, 1981; Rabbitt and Vyas, 1970) grounds. An alternative model for the way in which people equivocate between speed and accuracy assumes that they must actively vary response speed to discover just how fast they can respond before they begin to make intolerable numbers of errors (Rabbit, 1980, 1981; Rabbit and Vyas, 1970). This model accounts for particular aspects of changes of CRT with practice which others, such as that by Newell and Rosenbloom (1981), have not yet considered. Mean CRT reduces dramatically with practice, not because people learn to make faster responses, but because they learn to make more fast responses and fewer slow responses.

Table 3 presents distributions of CRTs for the first and last sessions of 30 000 responses produced by a volunteer on an easy four-choice serial CRT task. Practice reduced mean RT from 531 msec to 379 msec but did not drastically alter the speed of the fastest responses produced. The volunteer reduced her mean RT by reducing the trial-to-trial variance (148–73 msec) and the skew of her RT distributions, rather than by shifting her entire RT distributions along the RT axis.

Figure 1 shows pooled distributions of CRTs produced by 40 volunteers during 2 000 experimental trials on an equiprobable four-choice, serial,

Table 3. Response latency distributions for the first and last day made by a single volunteer highly practised (30 000 responses in total) at an easy, continuous, self-paced serial four-choice CRT task

RT interval (msec)	Responses: 1–1689 number of correct responses	Responses: 28093–30000 numer of correct responses
240–279	0	26
280–319	5	187
320–359	29	448
360–399	92	411
400–439	229	219
440–479	320	103
480–519	304	42
520–559	214	19
560–599	118	6
600–639	94	7
640–679	60	4
680–719	43	1
720–759	29	1
760–799	22	0
800–839	25	1
840–879	15	3
880–919	7	1
920–959	13	2
960–999	4	0
1000+	2	0
Total correct	1625	1481
Total errors	32	213
Deleted responses following errors	32	213
Total	1689	1907

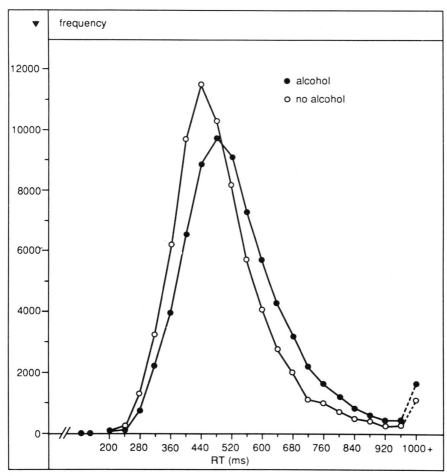

Figure 1. Pooled distributions of correct responses in a continuous, serial, four-choice response task obtained from each of 40 volunteers after ingesting either 0 ml or 1 ml alcohol per kg body weight.

self-paced CRT task under 0 ml and 1 ml alcohol per kg body weight. Alcohol increased mean correct CRT from 522 msec to 562 msec, medians from 503 msec to 540 msec, and standard deviations from 128 msec to 149 msec. Mean error CRT increased from 487 msec to 520 msec, median error CRT from 469 msec to 502 msec, and standard deviations from 116 msec to 136 msec. It can be seen that alcohol, like practice, shifts means and medians by altering the skew and variance of RT distributions. In these cases median or mean RTs are second-order indices of changes of efficiency. To assess true changes in the limits of efficiency of any task it is necessary to define the relationship between maximum speed and accuracy by computing the speed-accuracy trade-off functions (SATOF) (Pachella and Pew, 1968; Pew, 1969; Rabbit and Vyas, 1970; Schouten and Bekker, 1967).

Figure 2 shows SATOFs computed from pooled distributions of error and correct RTs made by volunteers under the alcohol and no alcohol conditions. We see that alcohol does indeed reduce the maximum speed at which people can respond without making errors, and so alters the limits of performance which they can attain. On its own, this finding would be consistent with the idea that alcohol reduces CNS efficiency in some global way, such as by altering neural signal-to-noise ratios and thereby increasing the average sampling time necessary to discriminate between events. Nevertheless, the problem still remains that the changes in RT distributions do not reflect

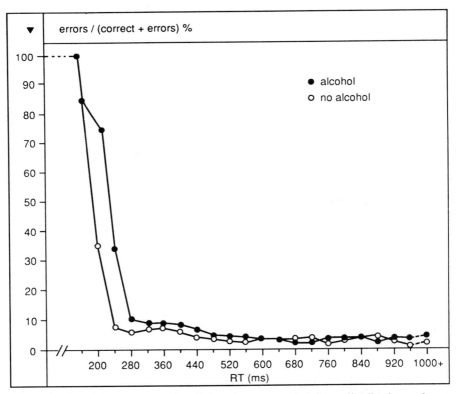

Figure 2. Speed–accuracy, trade-off functions computed from distributions of error and correct RTs for 2000 responces in a continuous, serial, four-choice response task made by each of 40 volunteers after ingesting either 0 ml or 1 ml alcohol per kg body weight.

changes of SATOF in any direct way. Volunteers showed only a small but insignificant increase of error rate in the alcohol sessions (4.97% vs. 4.14%). We might suppose that accuracy under alcohol was preserved by a corresponding shift of RT distributions to maintain accuracy. But a comparison of Figures 1 and 2 makes it clear that this was not the only, and perhaps not the most marked effect of alcohol. Speed was traded off against accuracy only over the narrow band of CRTs between 200 msec and 320 msec, and the most marked effects of alcohol were not to reduce the number of 'risky' responses transgressing the shifted SATOF, but rather to greatly increase the number of 'cautious' responses slower than 360 msec (Figure 1). It seems likely that alcohol does not merely alter the lower limit of accurate performance, but also alters the precision of the adaptation which people make to accommodate to changes in that limit.

These results emphasize that two distinct classes of satisfactory models for the cognitive operations underlying CRT may be based on two quite distinct assumptions: one class may be described as 'passive' models. An excellent exemplar is described by Laming (this volume). In such a model, parameters which determine the mean and variance of times taken for a random-walk process to reach a decision criterion may be adjusted, as by trial and error computer simulation (Bishop and Rabbitt, in preparation) so as to mimic the changes in mean CRT, in SATOFs and in the skew and variance in distributions of correct and error CRTs observed when volunteers experience practice, alcohol, or other conditions which alter their performance efficiency. A further step would be to identify these parameters in terms of plausible neural mechanisms which may be affected by these variables.

An alternative assumption is that people actively control their performance in continuous, serial CRT tasks to obey instructions to respond as fast and as accurately as they can. Volunteers can only fulfil these ambiguous instructions by responding increasingly quickly until they begin to transgress their SATOF, and sooner or later an error occurs. People detect most of the errors they make (Rabbitt, 1966, 1968). Thus, errors can provide feedback which allows people to slow their response speed and thus return, for one or more successive responses, to slower 'safe' CRT bands at which errors do not occur. They then again begin the process of speeding up their responses to track the current position of their SATOF, so as to find and learn the position of the narrow time window within which their responses may be optimally placed in order to fulfil experimental instructions to maximize both speed and accuracy (Rabbitt, 1980, Rabbit and Vyas, 1970). Consistent with this idea are demonstrations that RTs immediately preceding errors are faster than for other correct responses (Laming, this volume) and that CRTs immediately following an error are typically very slow (Rabbitt, 1970).

The limits of efficiency within which performance can be actively controlled in this way will be set by three distinct parameters. One of these, the slope of the SATOF, is directly related to the information processing rate. A second parameter is the reliability of detecting errors, without which there will be no feedback to identify the lower limit of the optimal time window within which responses should be placed. The third parameter is the efficiency of time estimation and temporal control of response speed. A coarsening of temporal control of responses will increase the minimum temporal steps used to track the SATOF, thus increasing both the number of avoidable fast errors and the trial-to-trial variance in CRT (Rabbitt, 1980, 1981; Rabbitt and Vyas, 1970).

Within the context of this active tracking model for maintenance of speed and accuracy, alcohol may reduce efficiency by degrading any or all of these parameters of performance. As we have seen, alcohol may impair performance by reducing the rate of information processing and so shifting the SATOF. But alcohol may also impair the distinct processes of error detection and of time estimation and temporal control of responses, which may, in practice, covary with the information processing rate, but which have not yet been directly related to the information processing rate in terms of any functional model of performance.

It is also noteworthy that active models of this kind must assume the existence of an hierarchical system with at least two levels. First there is a set of lower order processes, such as signal detection and identification, error detection, accurate time estimation, and temporal control of response production. These are subject to control by a higher order system which organizes performance so as to achieve a goal within the constraints which they determine. We have seen that alcohol may impair performance by perturbing one or more lower level processes which set limits to attainable efficiency. But on these assumptions alcohol may also affect the efficiency of higher order control processes, and so perturb performance in complex ways. One further detail of Maylor and Rabbitt's results is consistent with this interpretation. Table 4 shows mean CRTs for the four correct responses following each error

Table 4. Mean RTs (msec) for error (E) responses and correct (C) responses following errors made in a four-choice continuous, serial CRT task by 40 volunteers after ingesting either 0 ml or 1 ml alcohol per kg body weight

Trial-type (current trial in bold)	No alcohol	Alcohol
E	487	520
E**C**	572	641
EC**C**	533	575
ECC**C**	525	570
ECCC**C**	520	563

made in the alcohol and no alcohol conditions. There is not only a main effect of alcohol, slowing mean correct CRT, but also an interaction between the effects of alcohol and the size of the post-error slowing of CRT fist discussed by Rabbitt (1970). This exaggeration by alcohol of the brief disruption of performance following an error is consistent with the idea that alcohol does not only affect the efficiency with which higher order control processes in the cognitive system can organize performance to observe these limits.

Whether or not this or other active models for psychomotor performance prove useful in the long term, they serve an heuristic purpose in illustrating the general problem of identifying the level at which change or individual differences affect performance. This problem of level of description is well recognized in the neuropsychological literature, where models for alterations in performance are framed both in terms of lower level sensorimotor losses, and of perturbations of much higher level processes such as planning or organization which attain convincing, though often imprecise, ostensive definition in individual case studies. The simple point made here is that the problem of identifying all the possible levels of operation of a drug, a stressor, or condition such as age is as hard as any in the notoriously difficult neuropsychological literature. This is evident even in simple and direct tests or response speed and much more so when we test the ability to remember and recognize simple events.

Information Processing Rate in Memory Models

It might seem that the efficiency with which information can be stored in memory must depend on functional properties of the cognitive system quite different from those which mediate the speed and accuracy of decisions. In fact recent functional models of memory predict close relationships between information processing rate and memory capacity and duration. For example, Baddeley and Hitch (1974), Hulme (1984), and Hulme *et al.* (1984) have shown that in children and young adults memory span for words is directly related to measured articulation rate. For supraspan learning, the probability of recall is directly related to study time, and functional study time will obviously increase with information processing rate. Models such as that proposed by Craik and Lockhart (1972) directly related efficiency of long-term storage and retrieval to the 'depth' to which people can process items presented to them for later recognition or recall. Such models must predict that the depth of processing which can be accomplished during item presentation, and so the probability of subsequent recall, will vary directly with processing speed. Thus, these models predict that if conditions such as old age, drugs, or low IQ are associated with slow information processing rates, they should, for this reasons, also be associated with reduced memory efficiency.

Can all state-dependent changes of memory efficiency by regarded as second-ary consequences to reduced information processing rate?

Maylor and Rabbitt (in preparation) carried out an experiment in which 40 volunteers examined a series of 200 nouns presented to them one at a time on a computer-driven display to decide whether each had occurred earlier in the same series (old or new). These decisions were timed to within 10 msec. Sequences of words were made up to keep the probability of old and new words identical and constant on each trial throughout the run, with the obvious exception of the first word. Words were only repeated once, and repetitions occurred equally often (19 times) after intervals of 1, 4, 9, 19, and 49 intervening words. This was done to study changes in the speed and accuracy of recognition as a function of the passage of time and number of decisions intervening between the first and second appearance of repeated words. Volunteers classified different lists of words on separate days on which they were given either 0 ml or 1.0 ml alcohol per kg body weight. All factors were balanced.

Table 5 shows changes in recognition accuracy as a function of number of intervening items between the first and the subsequent presentation of a word. The probability of correct recognitions of repetitions of words fell with the interval between their successive appearances. Alcohol substantially reduced overall recognition probability and exaggerated the interval effect, apparently producing accelerated forgetting. These effects were not related to changes in the decision criterion with regard to old or new. As in all the experiments discussed above, alcohol also increased the time taken to make a decision about each word. Can this effect of alcohol on information loss be entirely accounted for by the concomitant effect on information processing rate?

Volunteers made the same decision (old or new) about each word in alcohol and no alcohol conditions. Thus, in one sense they were required to process the words to the same depth in both conditions. In the alcohol condition they took longer to make these decisions and so, in effect, took longer inspection times.

Table 5. Mean proportions of correct recognitions of repeated words in a series of 200 items, as a function of the number of intervening items between first and second appearance, after the ingestion of either 0 ml or 1 ml alcohol per kg body weight by 40 volunteers

	Number of intervening items				
	1	4	9	19	49
No alcohol	0.960	0.875	0.845	0.825	0.830
Alcohol	0.925	0.795	0.755	0.670	0.645

These extended inspection times were, however, obviously not adequate to maintain recognition accuracy.

This makes it difficult to explain the effects of alcohol on memory as a simple consequence of slowing of information processing. To translate this description into functional terms, we must postulate two separate factors, or even two separate systems, both of which are affected by alcohol. First, we may suppose that increased processing time does not compensate for reduced processing rate because both the 'quality' and amount of information processed is reduced by alcohol. Second, we may suppose that changes in the lower level parameter, information processing rate, are inadequately compensated by some higher order control system which adjusts inspection time to maintain the level of recognition accuracy. This system, perhaps, is also disabled by alcohol. Finally, we may suppose that alcohol—apart from affecting the rate, and so the amount, of information processing during initial classification of each item—also affects other quite different processes which determine the stability of memory traces, their rate of decay, and their vulnerability to interference. All these possible models require much more complex assumptions than a simple direct link between processing rate and memory efficiency.

Because Maylor and Rabbitt's experiment was not directly designed to explore correlations between processing speed and memory efficiency, it only incidentally reveals some of the logical complexities involved in interpreting these relationships. What kind of paradigm and data analysis will allow us to do this?

One promising new technique is to design experiments such that multivariate analyses are used to evaluate correlations between performance parameters. Rabbitt and Goward (1986) found that individual differences in mean CRT vary inversely with IQ test scores in populations of people aged 50–75 years. Mean CRT also increases with age, but this association disappears when age groups are matched for IQ test scores. Data gathered on a population of 2053 persons aged 50–92 years (Rabbitt *et al.*, in preparation), showed that performance on simple memory tasks, such as free recall of lists of 30 words, and cumulative learning of lists of 15 words, also varies with IQ test scores rather than with individual age. These data emphasize a question logically identical to that which we have discussed in relation to Maylor and Rabbitt's data: do people with high IQ test scores perform better on simple memory tests because they process information faster? Or do IQ tests pick up age changes in many different cognitive factors, and do these factors, apart from changes in speed, also contribute to a loss of efficiency at memory tasks?

Goward and Rabbitt (in preparation) attacked this question by requiring 76 volunteers aged 51–81 years to carry out two tasks involving study and subsequent recognition of lists of 32 nouns presented one at a time, in random order, on a computer-controlled display. In a so-called deep processing condition, they inspected the nouns to decide to which of two semantic categories they belonged (e.g., living vs. not living; manufactured vs. naturally occurring). In a so-called shallow processing condition, they decided whether or not each word contained a designated target letter (e.g., A or S). They signalled these decisions by pressing one or two response keys, and their RTs were measured to within 10 msec. Response probabilities were equal and constant across all trials. Word lists were made up so as to be categorizable in either condition, and these, with the order of testing, were balanced across volunteers.

Immediately after inspecting a list, volunteers scanned, one at a time, a further list in which the previous 32 words were randomly embedded among 32 distractors. They were asked to classify each word as new or old and these decisions were also timed and recorded.

The main findings were entirely consistent with the expectations from Craik and Lockhart's (1972) and Craik and Tulving's (1976) depth of processing models. Semantic classification took longer than letter detection, but recognition was more reliable after semantic than after surface processing. A new finding was that recognition of semantically processed items is much quicker, as well as more reliable, than recognition of items which have only been scanned to detect target letters.

The main interest of this experiment was, however, to try to assess the differential effects of age, IQ test scores, and information processing rate as factors determining the efficiency of recognition memory for words. The three age groups tested (50–59, 60–69, and 70–81 years) had been carefully matched for IQ test scores. A correlation between age and recognition efficiency was therefore neither expected nor obtained. From a multiple regression analysis run to compare age and categorization speed as predictors of recognition accuracy, categorization speed: $T = 3.48$, $P < 0.001$; and surface categorization speed gave significant prediction (semantic categorization speed: $T = 4.8$, $P < 0.001$), but chronological age gave no significant prediction when variance due to categorization speed had been partialled out. The same comparison was run comparing categorization speed and raw IQ test scores (AH 4 parts 1 and 2) as predictors of recognition accuracy. When variance due to IQ test scores had been partialled out, categorization speed did not predict recognition accuracy in either condition. But, even when categorization speed had been partialled out, IQ test score was a significant predictor ($T = -3.605$, $P < 0.5$). These results have been replicated with larger groups of volunteers in a more complex version of this task.

As people grow older their IQ test scores may decline, their information processing rate slows, and their recognition accuracy is reduced. Reduced information processing speed does nor seem, however, to be the master factor which mediates all other cognitive changes as some current theories of cognitive ageing would suggest (Salthouse, 1985). IQ test scores seem to pick up at least two different factors associated with recognition accuracy, and information processing speed not necessarily the more important.

These results also question recent suggestions by Band and Dearie (1982), Eysenck (1985). Hendricksen (1982), Jensen (1985), and Vernon (1983) that individual differences in IQ simply and directly reflect individual differences in information processing speed, which, in turn, directly reflect the efficiency of units in the CNS. It seems that there is more to being clever than being fast, and, in spite of Salthouse's (1985) thorough and critical review of the literature, there is more to being old than just being slow. In the context of the present discussion, the experiment illustrates a paradigm which we can use to directly attack the much more general question whether or not any particular psychopharmacological agent or state has its effect upon a wide range of apparently different cognitive tasks solely through its effect upon a single key parameter of performance—such as information processing rate. Or whether descriptions of changes in performance associated with agents or states rather require specification of changes in the operation of two or more distinct and separable variables.

Conclusions

The rate of information processing limits efficiency in many tasks and is therefore a very general, as well as very sensitive, index of changes of individual differences in cognitive performance. Differences in information processing rate are clearly one of the factors which are picked up by tests of general intelligence, and are also one of the most important factors contributing to changes in cognitive performance with advancing age (Salthouse, 1985). Information processing rate is also a sensitive index of the cognitive effects of drugs. But the experiments we have discussed make it clear that models which seek to explain all differences in cognitive performance associated with IQ, age, or drugs solely as second order effects of changes of information processing rate are too simple. They also question the general assumption that measures of mean CRT can be directly interpreted as indices of efficiency of fundamental neural processes.

Models for cognitive processes involved in recognition memory, digit span, efficiency of free recall, or rate of cumulative learning must incorporate decision speed as one important variable. Yet the results we have discussed suggest that decision speed is not a master variable controlling changes in all other performance parameters. This rejection of an attractive simple model is not merely a destructive exercise, since it focuses the questions we need to ask, produces some interesting leads for future research, and suggests new paradigms with which we may explore them.

References

Baddeley AD and Hitch GJ (1974) Working memory, in: Bower G (ed.) *The Psychology of Learning and Motivation* Vol. 8. New York: Academic Press.

Birren JE, Woods AM and Williams MV (1979) Speed of behaviour as an indicator of age changes and the integrity of the nervous system. In: Hoffmeister F and Müller C (eds) *Brain Function in Old Age*. pp. 10–44. Berlin: Springer.

Brand CR and Dearie IJ (1982) Intelligence and inspection time. In: Eysenck HJ (ed.) *A Model for Intelligence*. Berlin: Springer.

Craik FIM and Lockhart RS (1972) Levels of processing: A framework for memory research. *J. Verbal Learning Verbal Behaviour* **11**, 671–84.

Craik FIM and Tulving E (1975) Depth of processing and the retention of words in episodic memory. *J. Exp. Psych.: General* **104**, 268–94.

Eysenck JH (1985) The theory of intelligence and the psychophysiology of cognition In: Sternberg RJ (ed.) *Advances in Research in Intelligence. Vol. 3*. Hillsdale, New Jersey: Erlbaum.

Hendricksen AE (1982) The biological basis of intelligence Part I: Theory. In: Eysenck HJ (ed.) *A Model for Intelligence*. Berlin: Springer.

Hick. WE (1952) On the rate of gain of information. *Q. J. Exp. Psychol.* **4**, 11–26.

Hulme C (1984) Developmental differences in the effects of acoustic similarity on memory scan. *Dev. Psychol.* **20**, 650–7.

Hulme C, Thomson N, Muir C and Lawrence A (1984) Speech rate and the development of short-term memory. *J. Exp. Child Psychol.* **38**, 241–53.

Hyman R (1953) Stimulus information as a determinant of reaction time *J. Exp. Psychol.* **101**, 35–42.

Jensen AR (1985) The nature of black–white differences on various psychometric tests: Spearman's hypothesis *Behav. Brain Sci.* **8**, 193–219.

Newell A and Rosenbloom PS (1981) Mechanisms of skill acquisition and the law of practice. In: Anderson JR (ed.) *Cognitive Skills and their Acquisition*. Hillsdale, New Jersey: Erlbaum.

Neisser U (1963) Decision time without reaction time: Experiments in visual scanning. *Am. J. Psychol.* **76**, 376–85.

Pachella RG and Pew R (1968) Speed-accuracy trade-off in reaction times: Effect of discrete criterion times. *J. Exp. Psychol.* **76**, 19–24.

Pew RG (1969) The speed-accuracy operating characteristic. *Acta Psychol.* **30**, 16–26.

Rabbitt PMA (1966) Error correction time without external error signals. *Nature (London)*, **197** 1029–30.

Rabbitt PMA (1968) Three kinds of error-signalling responses in a serial choice task. *Q. J. Exp. Psychol.* **19**, 37–42.

Rabbitt PMA (1970) Psychological refractory delay and response-stimulus interval in serial choice-response tasks. *Acta Psychol.* **30**, 56–76.

Rabbitt PMA (1980) Control of responses in fast, continuous CRT tasks. In: Holding D (ed.) *Intelligence and Learning*. New York: Plenum Press.

Rabbitt PMA (1981) Cognitive psychology needs models for old age. In: Long J. and Baddeley AD (eds.) *Attention and Performance IX*. Hillsdale, New Jersey: Erlbaum.

Rabbitt PMA and Vyas SM (1970) An elementary preliminary taxonomy for some errors in laboratory choice-response tasks. *Acta Psychol.* **33**, 56–96.

Rabbitt PMA and Vyas SM (1977) Some errors of perceptual analysis in visual search can be detected and corrected *Q. J. Exp. Psychol.* **30**, 319–32.

Rabbitt PMA and Goward L (1986) Effects of age and raw I.Q. test scores on mean correct and mean error reaction times in serial choice tasks: A reply to Smith and Brewer. *Br. J. Psychol.* **77**, 69–73.

Salthouse TA (1985) *A Theory of Cognitive Ageing*. Amsterdam: North-Holland.

Schouten JF and Bekker JAM (1967) Reaction time and accuracy. *Acta Psychol.* **27**, 143–56.

Townsend JT and Ashby FG (1983) *Stochastic Modelling of Elementary Psychological Processes*. Cambridge: Cambridge University Press.

Vernon PA (1983) Speed of information processing and general intelligence. *Intelligence* **7**, 53–70.

Psychopharmacology and Reaction Time
Edited by I. Hindmarch, B. Aufdembrinke and H. Ott
© 1988 John Wiley & Sons Ltd

8

Reaction Time with Distractors: Some Possibilities for Drug Assessment

D. E. Broadbent

Department of Experimental Psychology, University of Oxford, Oxford, UK.

Abstract

This paper argues that studies of drug effects should measure a variety of different variables in a particular task in order to discriminate between various classes of drug. There is thus a need for short tests that can provide such measures, and one such test is introduced. It offers a number of alternative measures of attention; takes less than 15 minutes to administer; and detects different effects for different external variables, though not as yet pharmacological ones.

Introduction

When selecting tests for drug effects, it is highly desirable to use tasks that can be measured in a number of ways. Both from the armchair and from existing experiments, it is clear that different drugs will impair different aspects of neural function; hence, some aspects of behaviour will change while others will not. Gross tests, using some complex task that involves many neural subsystems, only measure the final success and may well miss the crucial deficit. This is particularly true because other aspects of neural function may change to compensate for the one that has been impaired. Such tests may therefore be insensitive. They also offer no insight into the way a drug is working that might be provided by detecting the particular subfunction that is changing.

Previous Work

Examples from past work include data on the effects of external noise. For instance, Smith (1985) has used a serial choice reaction task in which one signal occurs more frequently than the others. When noise is presented, there is an improvement in the speed of response to the probable signal. On the other hand, the speed of response to the improbable signals deteriorates. An average of the whole performance would have shown little, but the more subtle measure reveals that noise does indeed produce change.

Another aspect of performance that has been shown to be important for a number of environmental conditions is the distinction between the average speed at which a task is done and the frequency of brief periods of inefficiency, which are expressed as abnormally slow responses or errors. Jones (1983), for instance, used a serial choice reaction task, but with equal probability. The speed of response was also increased by keeping the fingers on the keys and thus minimizing movement; this may explain why the test was sensitive to noise levels lower than presented in earlier serial reaction tasks. There was no change in the average speed when noise was applied, but as in earlier studies there was an increase of errors.

Prolonged work tends to produce such gaps or errors after 10–15 minutes, and so to show the effects of noise it is necessary to continue the test for such a time. The average speed of work is only affected after much longer work periods. Sleeplessness also produced intermittent failures of performance, and again only after the task had been continued for a while (Wilkinson, 1963). As common sense would suggest, however, the effects of sleep loss are less pronounced when noise is present; the two conditions seem to cancel each other out.

Cancellation of this kind suggests at first sight the classic inverted U function relating performance to some general state of arousal, increased by stimulation (such as noise) and reduced by loss of sleep. If one is most efficient at moderate levels of arousal, it could well be that both sleeplessness and noise could impair efficiency, and yet their opposite effects on the state of arousal cancel each other out. Considering only such experiments, one could hold to a simple explanation of performance effects in terms of arousal.

On the other hand, some recent and still unpublished work in our laboratory used a serial reaction task to study the effects of three weeks' administration of diazepam at a dosage, recommended for severe anxiety, of 25 mg per day. There was no sign of an increase of errors, but rather of an improvement of accuracy accompanied by a slowing down of the average speed of response. Although diazepam impairs performance, just as do noise and sleeplessness, the effects are qualitatively different. There are other conditions which also produce this kind of effect; the point was first made by Mirsky and Rosvold (1960) and followed up by Broadbent (1971). Drugs and environmental conditions can be divided into two groups, one showing effects most easily on average speed and the other on response variability or error. Within each group, some effects cancelled each other out, as did noise and sleeplessness, but similar cancellations between groups were harder to find and inconsistent in direction. Tentatively, the group affecting average speed included time of day, the personality characteristic of introversion, alcohol, barbiturates, and diazepam. The second group included chlorpromazine and amphetamine, as well as noise and sleeplessness.

A rather different approach has led to a similar division of drug classes. Frowein (1981) used a complex reaction time task in which either the sensory display of information or the action needed for response could be made more difficult. The effect of changing the display was greater if the person had taken a barbiturate rather than amphetamine. In contrast, the effect of changing the response was greater if the person had taken amphetamine. Again, it is hard to resist the conclusion that the two drugs are affecting different mechanisms. If one accepts the additive factor logic of Sternberg (1969), as Sanders (1983) does, one could argue that the barbiturate alters an early stage of stimulus encoding, whereas amphetamine affects a response process. Even if one does not accept Sternberg's assumptions, however, the effects of barbiturates and amphetamine appear to be different.

Broadbent (1971) suggested that two mechanisms were involved in performance, one directly executing actions appropriate to the situation, while the other monitored and controlled the first. Thus, variables affecting one would cancel or reverse the effects of each other; but their impact on the other system would be less and inconsistent. There might be some impact, since the lower system would only show its effects if the monitoring control were relaxed; but this would apply which way the lower system was changing. This view and the one followed up by Sanders (1983) are not necessarily inconsistent; they may well both be true.

These two approaches show the desirability of measuring multiple aspects of performance. Yet there is often only limited time, and so it is preferable to get the measures in a relatively short test. In addition, the tests thus far discussed focus on the reaction to stimuli that appear without competition from distracting stimuli. In natural situations, the selective operations that determine the correct stimulus out of a total array are also important (Broadbent, 1982). These operations may take different forms, and again it is not clear that these forms will all be affected in the same way by a particular drug. It is therefore desirable to have a short test that measures a large variety of such attentional measures. The purpose of the present paper is to describe such a test.

The Technique Proposed

The basic technique is that of Eriksen and Eriksen (1974). The subject views a TV screen on which appear three fixation points, separated either by $0.5°$ or by $2°$. The subject knows that the central point is the only one that will be replaced by a reaction signal, and that the other locations can be ignored. The fixation points remain visible for 500 msec, and the central point is then replaced by either letter A or B. If A appears, a left-hand key must be pressed; and if B, the right-hand key. The irrelevant fixation points may be followed either by a pair of As, a pair of Bs, a pair of asterisks, or nothing. As soon as the reaction occurs, the fixation points reappear again with either a close or far spacing, and the cycle starts again.

Having completed a series of, say, 240 trials under these conditions, the subject is then given a fresh task. In this case only the two outer fixation points are used, spaced at the same intervals as in the previous case. The subject does not know which of them will be replaced by the reaction signal, which again may be A or B. Sometimes there will be nothing in the visual field except the reaction signal; sometimes there will be a distractor stimulus in the position of the other fixation point. Clearly, this cannot be a letter, as it sometimes was in the previous condition, because then the person would not know which letter was the reaction signal and which the distractor. In this case, therefore, the distractor is always a digit, so that the target is marked out by its membership of a category rather than its location. In contrast to the technique of Eriksen and Eriksen (1974), this condition is much more like the technique of Schneider and Shiffrin (1977), with the modification that a choice reaction rather than a signal detection is called for.

Characteristics of the Two Tasks

The two tasks are thus quite similar, but one has a known target location and the other has an unknown one. The difference between them corresponds to an important distinction between different kinds of selective attention (Broadbent, 1982; Kahneman and Treisman and 1984). Each task shows a number of effects that might be described as attention. Thus, the known location task shows the usual effect of Eriksen and Eriksen (1974), i.e., if the target is A and the distractors are B, or vice versa, the response is slower than when target and distractors agree, but only if they are close together. When there is a wide space between the target and the other letters, the distractors have no effect. Resistance to the effect of the distractor, even when close, might be described as selective attention, and so might the reduction of interference with spatial separation. Although there is on average no effect from the presence of an irrelevant asterisk, some subjects do slow down by comparison with the absence of distractors; and this again might be described as poor attention.

In the task with unknown location, a wide separation of target and distractor is more harmful than helpful; there is a compatibility effect, such that it is better for the A, which calls for a left-hand response, to appear on the left of the display rather than the right, and vice versa for the B. The ability to overcome this effect might be described as efficient attention, as might the ability to overcome the effect of spatial separation. In this task, just as in the one with known location, there may be distractors that point to neither reaction; in this case they produce a slowing down, but again the ability to resist this effect could be regarded as an index of effective attention.

Correlates of the Various Measures

In fact, any one of these effects from the one task fails to correlate with any of the effects from the other task. Thus, we appear to be measuring independent factors in the two varieties of selective attention.

By itself, this fact might simply mean that the various measurements are too crude to be valid. Individual measurements can, however, be related to external factors, showing that we are indeed measuring different functions, but that these are unrelated to each other. For example, the size of the Eriksen effect, the reduction in interference by spatial separation of target and distractors, is heavily affected by time of day. In six experiments, totalling over 120 subjects, we have found an overall reduction in the size of the effect in the afternoon, and no significant difference in the size of the effect in different experiments. The same relationship has been observed in studies in Sussex with a quite different subject population, experimenter, etc. Yet, other measures of attention, such as the difference between the two tasks, show no sign of such a relationship.

The difference between the two tasks is particularly interesting because of its link to the theoretical analyses of attention by Broadbent (1982). It is measuring the relative advantage produced by knowing the location of the reaction stimulus. That is, if one measures the difference, one is detecting the use of a strategy of selectively reacting to one location rather than a strategy of scanning the display widely to pick up instances of a category. The best established outside correlates of this measure are individual differences. It is related to obsessional personality, with those persons higher in obsessionality doing relatively better in the case of known location. It is also related in the opposite direction to the score on the Cognitive Failures Questionnaire (Broadbent *et al.*, 1982), with people who do well with an unknown location also reporting many slips or failures of performance in everyday life: forgetting where they have put things, failing to notice road signs, or dropping things. The two measures of individual differences act to some extent independently, each retaining a significant correlation when the other is cancelled out. One should not assume, however, that the measure of relative efficiency on the two tasks relates solely to lasting or permanent characteristics of the person, since it has been found that the level of anxiety exaggerates the effect of cognitive failures score. Such an interaction does not appear with, for example, the size of the Eriksen effect.

Thus, at least two of the scores measure some function detectable by links to outside variables. Others, such as the measure of compatibility effects, seem likely from the results of Frowein to be sensitive to outside variables, and there are a number of other potential candidates, such as the effects of those distractors that are unrelated to possible responses, response repetition effects, effects of repetition of the location of the unknown signal, and handedness. The two tasks can both be administered within 10–15 minutes, and the hope is that we shall be able to check for a large variety of functions in a reasonably short time. Thus far, no drugs have been used with the task, though we are at present analysing results with noise. We plan to examine some drugs in 1987.

References

Broadbent DE (1971) *Decision and Stress*. London: Academic Press.

Broadbent DE (1982) Task combination and selective intake of information. *Acta Psychol.* **50**, 253–90.

Broadbent DE, Copper PJ, Fitz Gerald PF and Parkes KR (1982) The Cognitive Failures Questionnaire (CFQ) and its correlates. *Br. J Clin. Psychol.* **21**, 1–16

Eriksen BA and Eriksen CW (1974) Effects of noise letters upon identification of target in a non-search task. *Percep. Psychophysics* **16**, 143–9.

Frowein HW (1981) Selective effects of barbiturate and amphetamine on information processing and response execution. *Acta Psychol.* **47**, 105–15.

Jones DM (1983) Loud noise and levels of control: a study of serial reaction. In: Rossi G (ed.) *Proceedings of the Fourth International Congress on Noise as a Public Health Problem.* pp. 809–817, Milan: Centro di Recherche e Studi Amplifon.

Kahneman D and Treisman A (1984) Changing views of attention and automaticity. In: Parasuraman R and Davies DR (eds.) *Varieties of Attention.* pp. 29–61, New York: Academic Press.

Mirsky AF and Rosvold HE (1960) The use of psychoactive drugs as a neuro-psychological tool in studies of attention in man. In: Uhr L and Miller JG (eds.) *Drugs and Behaviour.* pp. 375–392, New York.

Sanders AF (1983) Towards a model of stress and human performance. *Acta Psychol.* **53**, 61–97.

Schneider W and Shiffrin RM (1977) Controlled and automatic human information processing: I. Detection, search and attention. *Psychol. Rev.* **84**, 1–66.

Smith AP (1985) Noise, biased probability, and serial reaction. *Br. J. Psychol.* **76**, 89–96.

Sternberg S (1969) The discovery of processing stages: Extensions of Donder's method. In: Koster WG (ed.) *Attention and Performance* II. Amsterdam: North-Holland. (*Acta Psychologica* **30**, 276–315)

Wilkinson RT (1963) Interaction of noise with knowledge of results and sleep deprivation. *J. Exp. Psychol.* **63**, 332–7.

Psychopharmacology and Reaction Time
Edited by I. Hindmarch, B. Aufdembrinke and H. Ott
© 1988 John Wiley & Sons Ltd.

9

The Effects of Time of Day, Age, and Anxiety on a Choice Reaction Task

L. J. Frewer and I. Hindmarch

Human Psychopharmacology Research Unit, University of Leeds, Leeds, UK

Abstract

The effects of time of day, age and anxiety on a choice reaction time task (CRT) were examined. The task was designed such that two separate aspects of reaction time, the lift-off time (time taken to initiate a response following stimulus presentation) and movement time (time taken from initiation of response to completion of response) could be assessed independently. Three subject groups were included in the study: a young psychologically normal group ($n = 9$), a young anxious group ($n = 8$), and an elderly psychologically normal group. Assessments were made at two-hour intervals from 0800 to 2200 hours (a 'normal' diurnal period) for all subjects. It was found that performance on the CRT task was significantly impaired for both anxious and elderly normal subjects in comparison with the young normal group. Young anxious subjects exhibited an impairment attributable to the lift-off subcomponent of the task, whereas in the elderly normal group impairment was attributable to the movement subcomponent.

It was concluded that this result might reflect different response strategies within subject groups. No significant effects attributable to diurnal change within the young normal group were observed, although between-group differences in the diurnal performance curves were apparent. It was concluded that the division of the total CRT into subcomponents was relevant, since both the lift-off time and the movement time varied in a different way from the total CRT under the influence of the external variables of age, anxiety, and time of day.

Introduction

All choice reaction time (CRT) tasks used in psychopharmacological research

103

should give consistent results within drug-free subpopulations and be sensitive to appropriate external factors. This study was designed to examine the effects of time of day, anxiety, and age on a CRT task that has been successfully used to assess performance changes following psychotropic drugs (Hindmarch and Parrott, 1980; Hindmarch and Clyde, 1980).

CRT is one of the human assessment measures that exhibit a diurnal improvement of performance, paralleling temperature increments through the diurnal observation period (Mann *et al.*, 1975). A post-lunch dip, or midday increment in response latencies, has been observed in some studies (Blake, 1971). The theoretical explanation for diurnal changes is found in arousal theory (Monk, 1982). The CRT task described in this chapter should demonstrate such diurnal patterns of variation. The CRT latencies are expected to decrease through the diurnal period for a young psychologically normal subject group, i.e., subjects with no characteristics that may contribute to abnormal levels of arousal or atypical patterns of variation.

Anxiety can increase the response latencies of a CRT task (Kamin and Clark, 1957; Swantantra, 1981; Clyde, 1982). Anxious subjects are normally regarded as experiencing higher levels of arousal than non anxious subjects (Malmo, 1957; Cattell, 1966). Classically, performance impairment in anxious groups is explained by the application of the Yerkes–Dodson curve (Eysenck, 1969).

Many anxiety models attribute performance impairments in anxious groups to perceptual and other central factors rather than to peripheral or motor factors (Welford, 1973; Easterbrook, 1959; Broadbent, 1971; Hamilton, 1975, 1979). This suggests that any performance decrement in the anxious subject group would be predominant in the lift-off component rather than in the motor response component of the CRT task.

An interaction between time of day and anxiety may occur. If anxiety is associated with greater than optimal levels of arousal, maximum impairment should occur in the latter half of the diurnal period, when arousal is believed to be at a maximum. This obviously also implies that a typical diurnal variation actually occurs in the anxious group.

Increased response latencies have also been observed with increasing age. Welford (1977) noted that changes in the level of arousal with ageing do not lead to an increase of reaction time. Botwinnick (1973) reported that the increment in response latency in older subjects is apparently attributable to central decision processes rather than motor processes. Further support for this finding was offered by Surwillo (1963). Thus the lift-off component of the CRT task is more likely to be impaired in the elderly subject group than the pure motor component.

Finally, an interaction between time of day and age may be observed. Since diurnal variation is dependent on both physiological and psychological factors, both may contribute to the disentrainment of the rhythm, or an 'atypical' pattern of variation in elderly subjects. Disrupted sleeping patterns (Weitzman *et al.*, 1982), social changes, and physiological changes (Serio *et al.*, 1970) may all result in atypical patterns of diurnal variation. Wever (1973) observed desynchronization rhythms in all older subjects used in his isolated experimental sample compared with only 25% of the younger control group. However, it must be remembered that increased fatigue in an elderly subject group may also produce performance decrements.

To summarize, we propose that

1. Total CRT will exhibit a diurnal increase in response latencies for a young normal subject group.
2. A significant increase in CRT response latencies will be observed for both young anxious and elderly normal subjects when compared with young normal subjects.
3. The increased CRT response latency will be attributable to the lift-off time in the CRT task.
4. Differences in the observed diurnal performance curves will be found for both young anxious and elderly normal subjects when compared with young normal subjects, i.e., young anxious subjects will exhibit maximum impairment in the latter half of the diurnal period. Elderly subjects will exhibit an atypical diurnal curve, attributable to both exogenous and endogenous diurnal disentrainment, and increased levels of fatigue towards the end of the diurnal period.

Method and Procedure

Reaction time was measured on the Leeds Psychomotor Tester[*] (LPT), whose stimulus consists of one of six light sources turned on in random succession. The required response is a movement of the index finger from a resting position to a response button adjacent to the stimulus light.

The configuration and dimensions of the LPT are shown in Figure. 1. In operation, the LPT is placed on a flat surface some 50 cm from the subject's eyes. The preferred hand should be able to move freely over the surface of the test equipment. It is clenched with only the index finger extended, and this placed on the start button (A). The angle subtended between buttons B1 and B6 at button A is 120 deg, and so the subject can monitor all the stimulus lights (L1—L6) without undue head movements.

A random presentation of a series of stimulus lights can be initiated manually or on-line via a computer. The subject begins an experimental session with his finger on button A and responds to the presentation of a stimulus light (L1—L6) by moving his finger as quickly as possible from A to

---

[*] Details from Leeds Psychomotor Services, 2 Acomb Court, Front Street, Acomb, York, UK

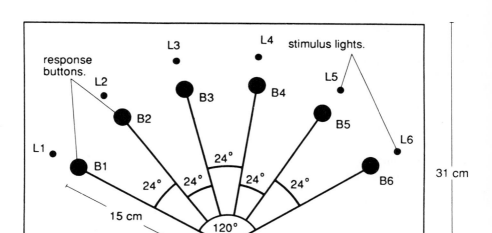

Figure 1. Configuration and dimensions of the CRT task from the Leeds Psychomotor Tester.

the appropriate B button. All buttons are 1 cm in diameter and are arranged at equal intervals of 24° about the arc of a circle centring on A. Each button (B1–B6) is at the same distance (15 cm) from start button A. All buttons are touch sensitive with no mechanical parts. The LPT measures the latency of the reaction to the stimulus light, i.e., the time between the illumination of one of the stimulus lights (L1–L6) and the touching of the appropriate button (B1–B6). The equipment separately measures the lift-off time between the illumination of one of the lights (L1–L6) and the movement of the finger from button A. The time taken to move from A to one of the B buttons (movement time) can be obtained by subtracting the lift-off time from the total reaction time.

Mean total reaction times are obtained from at least 25 presentations of stimulus lights, while sequential reaction times can be obtained from mean response times for consecutive sequences of fewer trials. The task requirements have been purposely kept simple, and no difficulties have been encountered in training subjects and using the LPT in experimental populations aged 3–90 years. All subjects are given pre-experimental training, but exposure to 100 stimulus presentations is sufficient to establish plateau reaction times in the majority of pre-trial situations. With the present configuration, constant since 1975, there seems to be no evidence that subjects decide where to move after they have left the start button. With response times of 350–700 msec in healthy psychologically normal populations aged 25–55 years, the motor reaction to the stimulus lights is almost reflex. Under these conditions we believe that the lift-off time represents the latency of processes other than motor execution and thus reflects aspects of the speed of stimulus recognition and response organization (e.g., Fitts, 1954; Kerr, 1973). Note, however, that the lifting off is itself a movement taking a finite time, and thus the actual lift-off reaction must contain some motor component.

Only male subjects were selected for this study so as to avoid any possible interactions with the menstrual cycle (Landauer, 1974).

There were three subject groups: a) a young normal groups ($n = 9$; mean age 23.2 years, range 22–25 years); b) a young anxious group ($n = 8$; mean age 23.5 years, range 23–25 years); and c) and elderly normal subject group ($n = 9$; mean age 63.4 years, range 58–68 years). All subjects were volunteers and in good physical health. The use of psychotropic drugs in the four weeks before the study precluded inclusion in the experiment.

Anxiety was rated with the Free Floating Anxiety Subscale (FFAS) of the Middlesex Hospital Questionnaire (Crown and Crisp, 1970). Subjects scoring eight points or more on the FFAS were allocated to the anxious group. This criterion has been used successfully by Hill *et al.* (1981). The mean FFAS score was 3.11 (range 0–5) for the young normal group, 10.37 (range 8–15) for the young anxious group, and 2.37 (range 0–6) for the elderly group.

The CRT task was actually part of a larger test battery, yet only the results of the CRT assessment are reported here. Ambient temperature and lighting were maintained constant in the test room throughout the diurnal period. Each subject was tested at two-hour intervals from 0800 to 2200 hours. On each occasion a mean of 25 CRT trials was collected. Subjects were instructed to avoid caffeine and alcohol on the test day itself. All subjects were permitted to follow their normal daily routine (within reason).

Results

Diurnal changes within the normal group

Total CRT latencies were split into lift-off time and movement time components. A single factor ANOVA with repeated measures was used to compare CRT response latencies within the young group. A least squares test was used to make an *a priori* comparison of means where a significant main effect indicated that this was appropriate.

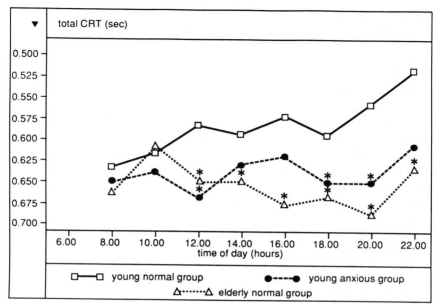

Figure 2. Mean total CRT response latencies plotted against time for young normal subjects, young anxious subjects, and elderly normal subjects. Asterisks above group means (for young anxious and elderly subject groups) indicate significant differences (P < 0·05) from the young normal group at specific times of day.

Total CRT

The mean total reaction time (in msec) plotted against time of day for all subject groups in illustrated in Figure 2. No significant main effect attributable to time was observed. The hypothesis of a diurnal decrease in response latency on total CRT was, therefore, not confirmed.

Lift-off time

The mean lift-off times, plotted against time of day for all subject groups, are illustrated in Figure 3. Again, no significant main effect attributable to time was observed. The hypothesis that there would be a diurnal decrease in lift-off response latencies in the normal group was, therefore, not confirmed.

Movement time

The mean movement times, plotted against time of day for all subject groups, is illustrated in Figure 4. A significant main effect attributable to time was observed ($F = 3.58$; d.f. = 7.56; $P < 0.0031$). *A priori* means comparisons indicated that the initial assessment at 0800 hours was significantly slower than the assessment at all other times apart from at 1800 and 2000 hours

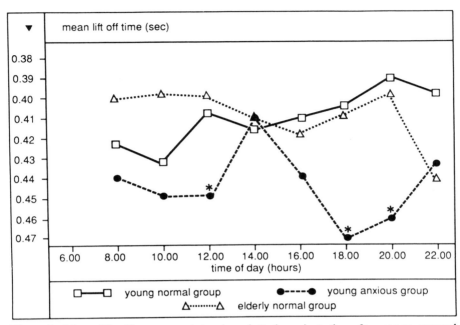

Figure 3. Mean lift-off response latencies plotted against time for young normal subjects, young anxious subjects, and elderly normal subjects. For explanation of symbols, see Figure 2.

($P < 0.05$), and that the 2000 assessment was significantly slower than the 1200 and 1600 hours assessment ($P < 0.05$). That is, the movement reaction times were fastest in the afternoon (1200–1600 hours) with an additional increase in the final tests. Although the hypothesis of a diurnal change cannot be rejected, the diurnal curve does not exhibit the expected pattern of decrease in latency, and so cannot be said to exhibit a typical pattern of diurnal variation.

Between-group comparisons

The young normal group was compared with the young anxious group and the elderly normal group. A split plot ANOVA with repeated measures was performed for each comparison, total CRT, lift-off time, and movement time. *A priori* comparisons for significant main effects were performed using a least means square comparison. Between-group comparisons were performed using the confidence interval for difference among planned orthogonal comparisons. (Kirk, 1968).

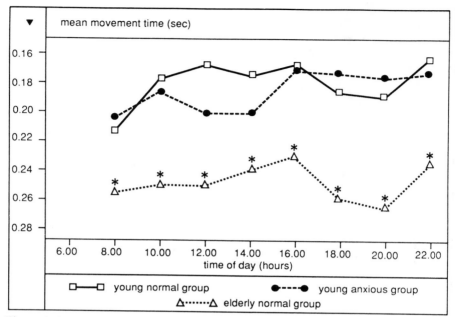

Figure 4. Mean movement response latencies plotted against time for young normal subjects, young anxious subjects, and elderly normal subjects. For explanation of symbols, see Figure 2.

Total CRT

The group means plotted against time of day are found in Figure 2. The comparison between the young normal group and the young anxious group revealed a significant main effect attributable to the intergroup differences ($F = 22.97$; d.f. $= 1.105$; $P < 0.0001$). Anxious subjects exhibited significantly longer response latencies on the total CRT assessment at 1200, 1800, and 2000 hours ($P < 0.05$). The hypothesis that anxious subjects exhibit significantly slower response latencies than normal subjects was therefore confirmed. Furthermore, these differences tended to occur in the latter part of the diurnal period. No significant main effect was attributable to time of day, as follows from the first analysis, nor was there any significant interaction between time of day and groups. The hypothesis that there would be an interaction between time of day and groups was not confirmed.

A significant main effect attributable to differences between groups was also observed in the comparison between young normal subjects and elderly normal subjects ($F = 33.97$; d.f. $= 1.105$; $P < 0.001$) Significant between-group differences occurred at all times, including the 1200 hour assessment ($P < 0.05$). The hypothesis that elderly subjects would exhibit significantly slower total CRT latencies was confirmed. These differences tended to occur in the latter half of the diurnal period. Yet no significant main effects were attributed to time of day, nor was there a significant interaction between time of day and groups.

Lift-off time

The group means plotted against time of day are illustrated in Figure 3.

The comparison between the young normal and young anxious subject groups revealed a significant main effect attributable to group differences ($F = 24.78$; d.f. = 1.105; $P < 0.01$). These between-group differences were significant at the 1200, 1800, and 2000 hour assessments showing that anxious subjects exhibit significantly slower lift-off response latencies than the normal group. No significant main effect was attributable to time, nor was there a significant interaction between time of day and group differences.

By contrast, the comparison of the lift-off response latencies of the young normal and elderly normal subjects indicated that there was no significant main effect attributable to time of day. The hypothesis that impaired CRT latency in the elderly group would be located in the lift-off component of the task was rejected. Furthermore, there was neither a significant main effect attributable to time nor a significant interaction between time and group.

Movement time

A contrasting pattern of results was observed for the movement component of the CRT task. The comparison of the young normal and young anxious subjects indicated that there were neither significant main effects nor a significant interaction between group and time. The hypothesis that anxious subjects would exhibit an impaired movement time was not confirmed. Furthermore, neither anxiety nor time of day affected the movement component. The comparison of young normal and elderly anxious subjects, however, indicated a significant main effect attributable to time ($F = 135.39$; d.f. = 1.105; $P < 0.0001$). A significant between-group difference was observed at all times of the diurnal period ($P < 0.05$). Again, no significant main effect was attributable to time, nor was there a significant interaction between time of day and groups.

In summary, it was found that CRT performance was impaired by both age and anxiety, as expected. Total reaction time results indicate that the impairment occurred towards the latter half of the diurnal period for both the anxious and elderly groups. Further analysis of the lift-off and movement components indicated that the impairment was selective within each group. Impairment within the young anxious group was attributable to the lift-off time, whereas in the elderly group it was attributable to the movement component. No statistically significant diurnal changes representative of typical diurnal performance changes were observed, nor were there any significant interactions between group differences and time of day.

Discussion

No significant diurnal decrease in CRT response latencies was observed within the young normal group, although response times for total CRT and the lift-off time tended to increase over the diurnal period. The failure to replicate earlier findings (Blake, 1971) could be attributable to the magnitude of the effect observed with small subject populations and the brief periods of testing, rather than to problems within the CRT test itself. Within the anxious group, a significant impairment of CRT performance was observed. A similar pattern of impairment of total CRT was observed in the elderly group. An analysis of the subcomponents of each task revealed that the performance decrement in the anxious group was primarily attributable to the lift-off component of the CRT. This suggests that decision processes leading to the lift-off response and its motor component are affected by anxiety. No significant increase of the lift-off time was observed for the elderly group.

If age-related CRT increases are mainly due to central interpretative factors, then it appears that any response latencies deriving from such factors must have been assessed within the movement time subcomponent of the task. One possible interpretation of these findings is that different response strategies were being used by the anxious and elderly group. The young anxious subjects might have selected responses before initiating the motor action, whereas the opposite could be true for the elderly subjects. This may be attributable to differences of motivation between the two groups, older subjects being more prone to respond before stimulus exposure.

We would argue, however, that this is not the case. There is evidence to suggest that the cognitive components of CRT are separate from the motor components (Fitts, 1954; Kerr, 1973; Schmidt *et al.*, 1984). It seems improbable that the relationship between the two components was changed in the sense that older subjects adopted a more risky strategy, since the elderly generally tend to adopt more conservative strategies.

An alternative conclusion is that the increased CRT response latency observed in the elderly is primarily motor in origin. Whilst diurnal changes within the normal group were not significant, it is still important to examine comparative performance effects within the anxious and elderly groups at specific times of day. Anxious subjects exhibited a significant performance impairment at 1200, 1800, and 2000 hours. This pattern of impairment was observed in the total CRT and the lift-off time. This supports that notion that the performance impairment in the anxious group is maximum when arousal is maximum the 1400 hour performance improvement might reflect an inverted post-lunch dip, since the post-lunch dip in the diurnal performance curve is normally attributed to a subjective decrement of alertness (Blake, 1971).

The elderly group exhibited an increase total CRT in the latter half of the diurnal period which was attributable to the movement component. Since the significant effects on the movement component were unrelated to time of day, this cannot be attributed to between-group differences in fatigue. As far the lift-off component is concerned, elderly subjects tended to be faster than the young normal subjects at the beginning fo the diurnal period; this difference explains why the total CRT response latencies of the elderly subjects were not significantly slower at all observation times. Some flattening of the diurnal performance curve may be indicated, but further research must be done to clarify this.

In conclusion, it appears that the division of the total CRT into the subcomponents of lift-off and movement time permits the experimental examination of the components of reaction time that vary, under the influence of external variables, in a different way to the changes in total reaction time.

References

Blake MFJ (1971) Temperament and time of day. In: Colquhoun WP (ed.) *Biological Rhythms and Human Performance* pp. 109–148. London: Academic Press.
Botwinnick J (1973) *Ageing and Behaviour.* New York: Springer.
Broadbent DE (1971) *Decision and Stress.* New York: Academic Press.
Cattell RB (1966) Anxiety and motivation; theory and crucial experiments. In: Spielberger CD (ed.) *Anxiety and Behavior.* New York: Academic Press.
Clyde CA (1982) *The Relationship between Personality and the Effects of Benzodiazepine Derivatives on Psychomotor Performance.* University of Leeds: Doctoral thesis.
Crown S and Crisp DH (1970) Manual of the Middlesex Hospital Questionnaire. *Psychological Test Publications.* Barnstable: Devon.
Easterbrook JA (1959) The effect of emotion on cue utilisation and the organization of behaviour. *Psychol. Rev.* **66**, 183–201.
Eysenck HJ (1969) Psychological aspects of anxiety. In: Lader MH (ed.) *Studies of Anxiety.* Ashford, Kent: Headly Brothers Ltd.
Fitts PM (1954) The information capacity of the human motor system in controlling the amplitude of movement. *J. Exp. Psychol.* **47**, 381–91.
Hamilton V (1975) Socialization anxiety and information processing: A capacity model of anxiety-induced performance deficits. In: Sarason IG and Spielberger CD (eds.) *Stress and Anxiety*, Vol. II New York: Wiley.
Hamilton V (1979) Information processing aspects of neurotic anxiety and the schizophrenias. In: Hamilton V and Warburton D (eds.) *Information Processing Approach.* London: Wiley.
Hill AJ, Walsh RD and Hindmarch I (1981) Tolerability of nocturnal doses of clobazam in anxious patients in general practice. *R. Soc. Med. International Congress and Symposium Series* **43**, 133–140.
Hindmarch I. and Clyde CA, (1980) A preliminary investigation of the effects of a 1,4 benodiazepine derivative (HR 158) on subjective aspects of sleep and objective measures of early morning performance. *Drugs Exp. Clin., Res.* **2**, 61–70.
Hindmarch I and Parrott AC (1980) The effects of combined sedative and anxiolytic preparations on subjective aspects of sleep and objective measures of arousal and performance the morning following nocturnal treatment. II: Repeated Doses. *Arzneimittelforschung* **30**, 1167–70.

Kamin LJ and Clarke KW (1957) Taylor Scale and Reaction Time *J. Abnorm. Soc. Psychol.* **54**, 262–63.

Kerr R (1973), Movement time in an underwater environment *J. Mot. Behav.* **5**[3], 175–8.

Kirk RE (1968) *Experimental Design, Procedures for the Behavioural Sciences.* California: Wadsworth Publishing Company.

Landauer AA (1974) Choice decision time and the menstrual cycle. *Practitioner I.* **213**, 703–6.

Malmo RB (1957) Anxiety and behavioural arousal. *Psychol. Rev.* **64**, 276–87.

Mann M, Ratenfranz J and Aschoff J (1975) Untersuchung zur Tagesperiodik der Reaktionszeit bei Nachtarbeit. I. Die Phasenlage des positiven Scheitel-Wertes and Einflüß des Schlafs auf die Schwingungsbreite. *Int. Arch. Arbeitsmed.* **29**, 159–74.

Monk TM (1982) The arousal model of time of day effects in human performance efficiency. *Chronobiologia* **9**, 49–54.

Schmidt KH, Kleinbeck Y and Brockman W (1984) Motivational control of motor performance by goal setting in a dual task situation. *Psychol. Res.* **46**, 129–41.

Serio M, Piolanti P, Romano S, De Magistris L and Guisti G (1970) The circadian rhythm of plasma cortisol in subjects over 70 years of age. *J. Gernontol.*, **25**, 95–7.

Surwillo WW (1963) The relation of simple response time to brain wave frequency and the effect of age. *Electroencephalogr. Clin. Neurophysiol.* **15**, 105–14.

Swantantra J (1981) Anxiety in relation to task complexity. *Indian J. Clin. Psychol.* **8**, 147–9.

Weitzman ED, Moline MG, Czeislev CA and Zimmermann JC (1982) Chronobiology of ageing: Temperature, sleep-wave rhythms and entrainment. *Neurobiol. Aging* **13**, 297–309.

Welford AT (1973) Stress and performance. *Ergonomics* **16**, 567–80.

Welford AT (1977) Motor performance. In: Birren JE and Schaie KW (eds.) *Handbook of the Psychology of Ageing* New York: Van Nostrand Reinhold

Wever R (1973) The meaning of circadian cyclicity with regard to ageing in man. *Verh. Dtsch. Ges. Pathol.* **59**, 160–80.

Psychopharmacology and Reaction Time
Edited by I. Hindmarch, B. Aufdembrinke and H. Ott
© 1988 John Wiley & Sons Ltd.

10

Relative Advantages and Disadvantages of Various Performance Measures in the Assessment of Psychotropic Drug Effects

A. F. Sanders

Institute of Psychology. RWTH, Aachen, FRG

Abstract

This paper presents a brief review of some current performance measures and their background with respect to the evaluation of the effects of psychotropic drugs on human performance.

The starting point is the notion that measures should ultimately help predict effects on real life performance, such as driving or the operation and supervision of machines. Yet it is difficult and often impossible to obtain direct or even indirect measures of real life performance. The feasibility of constructing a standard set of tasks is briefly considered, and some approaches are reviewed.

The vast majority of tasks can be divided into measures of either reaction time or of accuracy. Both have their advantages and disadvantages, but time measures clearly offer more opportunities for a finegrained analysis. In general, however, a choice ought not be made between the two types of test. Rather, more sophisticated composite measures should be elaborated.

Introduction

A major aim of psychotropic drug research is to describe detailed patterns of effects and side-effects of the various drugs on human performance, as well as on behaviour in general. Research into biochemical and physiological effects—although highly valuable in itself—tells us relatively little about performance, and nothing about the selective effects produced after low dosages. Results of animal studies are also of limited value for the prediction of effects on human skills. A good example are the animal studies into the behavioural effects of ACTH (4–10) that had consistently shown a decrease in the speed of the extinction of conditioned responses. This suggested that ACTH (4–10) could affect memory, and for some time pharmacologists actually hoped that a 'learning pill' had been discovered. Yet subsequent studies with human subjects failed to show any effect on traditional verbal learning and retention. In addition, there was no effect on the reactive inhibition component of a massed practiced sensorimotor skill. Hence, it was concluded that ACTH (4–10) promotes performance, but through motivation and not through learning (Gaillard and Varey, 1979).

Research Methods

When assessing the effects of drugs on human performance, it is not enough to use some random sample of laboratory performance tasks (Hindmarch, 1980). The basic interest focuses on aspects of efficiency and the risks of accidents in everyday life. A typical example, and one that enjoys considerable popularity (e.g., O'Hanlon and de Gier, 1986), is traffic safety; but industrial safety and the risks of household accidents are equally important.

A major and well-recognized problem is that it is usually impossible or impractical to assess drug effects—but also effects of stressors such as sleep loss, noise, and heat—on performance in everyday life. Exceptions can be found in highly specific tasks and homogeneous work situations, where it is possible to make analyses on the basis of video pictures or to measure performance in actual practice. Typing (Shaffer, 1973) and piano playing (Shaffer, 1981) are good examples of skills that allow a finegrained analysis.

Although the limits of application of video techniques have still to be assessed adequately—in particular with regard to recent developments in the acquisition and processing of materials—it is improbable that this technique can be widely applied.

Moreover, epidemiological surveys are limited to more or less standard conditions, such as alcohol and driving (Borkenstein *et al.*, 1964) and, more recently, prolonged driving and effects of time of day (Harris, 1977). Such effects can be studied under standard driving conditions as observed in bus and lorry drivers.

Another possibility is the use of simulation. This has increasingly good prospects, given the rapid advances of computer science. At present there are computer-based simulations of complete tasks and sophisticated means of on-line data reduction in near real life conditions. A good example of the latter are experimental cars which permit actual on-the-road testing. For instance, Riemersma *et al.*, (1977) studied the effects of prolonged night driving, and O'Hanlon *et al.* (1982) more recently studied the effects of diazepam in on-the-road tests. Although such tests never fail to give the impression that they correspond to real life, there are in fact various limitations, including the prevention of accidents at all costs, usually a restricted set of measures, and the untypical motivational state of the subjects. Since the effects of most psychotropic drugs probably have a strong influence on motivation, this last limitation may be particularly serious.

Full task simulation is the next best. It is a valuable tool, but only if the simulator has been validated. Many simulators are claimed to test psychomotor abilities, say, in traffic, but without proper empirical underpinning. As I have pointed out elsewhere (Sanders, 1976), the problem with unvalidated simulators is that they neither advance a theory nor represent real life situations, and therefore the results do not really add to our knowledge.

The validation of simulators is a complex endeavour but certainly not altogether impossible, as shown in the work of Truyens and Schuffel (1978) and Blaauw (1977) on TNO simulators of ship manoeuvring and car driving. The validation method that was applied in both cases involved the simulation of a well-controlled and specific real life situation, e.g., manoeuvring a vessel through a narrow passage or approaching a difficult road crossing, and the correlation of behavioural actions in real life and the simulation. In the case of ship manoeuvring the results were very satisfactory: high correlations were observed between simulated and actual responses on a number of system parameters. Car driving simulation is as yet much less satisfactory, probably because of the enormous problems in providing the proper feedback of movement and force.

When measuring performance on simulators or in real life, a major issue is that the results usually give only rough indications that are highly task specific and hard to analyse. Again, there are exceptions, such as typing, but the lack of a detailed analysis is usually the price paid for opting for real life situations. In contrast, results can be better analysed in the laboratory, but such a set up cannot be extrapolated without further course to real life. Gopher and Sanders (1984) have recently proposed the principle of back-to-back study. In this research strategy, inferences from laboratory tasks are subsequently tested in the actual field or on a good simulator.

The systematic application of back-to-back studies could show where and when laboratory tests are predictive and, more importantly perhaps, why laboratory tests are sometimes not predictive. The comparison between high-speed perceptual motor skills such as typing and piano playing, and the slow responding in laboratory tests, as exemplified by the psychological refractory period (Shaffer, 1975, 1980) may serve as a case in point. I am convinced that future tests of drug effects on performance and behaviour will consist of a combination of standardized sets of laboratory performance tasks and questionnaires. The laboratory test has probably the unique advantage of a bridge position between real life and biochemical and physiological aspects of investigation. As argued above, the contacts with real life might be accomplished through the back-to-back approach. In addition, the more restricted and abstract setting of the laboratory task is more appropriate in the search for biochemical and physiological correlates of performance. The developments in the research into event-related potentials (e.g., Näätänen *et al.*, 1982) are a good example.

Towards a Set of Standard Tasks

A major issue for the investigator is to decide what laboratory tasks to use or, better perhaps, how to develop tasks that are both ecologically relevant and clearly coupled to certain mental functions. Moreover, not only must a set of standard tasks be developed, but also suitable measures have to be selected.

The need and relevance of such an endeavour is well recognized, although there are divergent opinions about its actual feasibility. Fleishman (1982) has recently listed some of the major advantages of standardized tasks in combination with a more generally accepted task taxonomy. These advantages include application to job analysis, personnel selection and training, and anchors for the evaluation of environmental and organismic factors. The major concern of Fleishman and coworkers was to define abilities by way of factor analysis. This had led to a battery of tasks, each of which is thought to be typical for a certain mental ability. For example, 'finger dexterity,' 'multi-limb co-ordination,' and 'dynamic flexibility' would constitute different motor abilities measured by different tests. In several major projects, Fleishman and coworkers found selective effects of drugs (e.g., scopolamine) and noise on some tasks of the battery (Elkin *et al.*, 1965; Baker *et al.*, 1967; Theologus *et al.*, 1974). In addition, Fleishman and co-workers have claimed that their tests are a good prediction of real life skills.

Yet as far as I am aware, the Fleishman approach has not found wide acceptance; this is probably due to its largely empirical character. Instead, various other attempts are being developed on the basis of some conceptual theoretical framework, although not very rigorously. Examples are the criterion-set task battery (Shingledecker, 1984) of Wright-Patterson and the '10 tasks' of TNO. The former relies upon multiple resource notions (e.g., Wickens, 1984), whereas the '10 tasks' are somewhat more eclectic but have bearings on linear stage analysis (e.g., Sanders, 1983). Note that these more recent attempts have been much less validated empirically than the Fleishman battery. It remains to be seen to what extent the results of the various approaches converge to a common conclusion concerning a finite number of 'radicals' in human performance, i.e., abilities, resource types, processing stages. The question is ultimately whether such components are basic constraints and generalise from laboratory to real life. The concept of components would still be useful when complemented by a strategic executive—at least if the executive is limited to a finite and describable number of strategies. An alternative is that each new task—or even variations of the same task

—constitutes a new 'whole', qualitatively different from anything else. In the extreme case (Neisser, 1976), the prospects for a systematic experimental psychology—and anything more than a rudimentary brain and behaviour theory—look rather bleak.

The alternative extreme considers only a finite number of abilities and comes close to a classical faculty notion. It excludes integrative strategic principles in human performance. It is clear by now that this alternative is wrong. Strategies are relevant and cannot be ignored. The question is rather to what extent strategic freedom is subject to constraints, as set by abilities and a restricted number of possible strategic approaches. Thus, strategies could have some degree of control over the modules required by a certain task without controlling the contents of the modules in anything more than evident ways. This does not imply that the modules are fully static and unchangeable. On the contrary, they are likely to change with practice or disuse. Practice in a given task has often been thought to change the relative weighting of the modules (Fleishman, 1985; Heuer, 1984). In addition, the contents of the structure of the modules are likely to develop with age and skill acquisition. It is, of course, hoped that laboratory experimentation will shed some light on the basic modules, the types of available strategies, and the integration of strategy and processing constraints.

Time and Accuracy Measures

At this point the discussion may return to the type of laboratory tests that could be fruitful as elements of a standardized battery and, from there, to the major theme of what measures should be used in drug research. In fact a discussion of the measures might provide some concrete proposals, since the measures to a large extent dictate what information can be obtained. It is then generally recognized that we basically have only two behavioural measures, namely time and judgement. All measures are derived from these two basics inasmuch as they are either chronometric or consist of a percentage of correct responses or ratings. For example, psychophysics and its derived measures of signal detection and recognition are based upon judgement. Much in the same way, error scores in tracking and forgetting or errors resulting from an overload of task demands are basically 'percentages correct'. Finally, all subjective judgements in terms of rating or rank ordering are based upon this principle.

The idea behind error scores in the measurement of performance is to bring the subject to the very limits of his performance, thus preventing perfect task execution while at the same time giving him the chance to make correct responses. In fact, ceiling and floor effects are a constant danger to all error-based measures. Ideally, correct responses should be within the 20–80% range, since extreme values usually make a correct interpretation difficult.

Transformations of the extremes are usually not very helpful since they bring about strong effects of small accuracy changes.

Another major problem for accuracy measures is that they can by definition only be obtained for a relatively large number of trials. This in turn means that a finegrained analysis is usually impossible. An interesting example is provided in the application of signal detection measures, where some 50–100 trials are needed to calculate the relevant measures of β and d'. A major assumption is that there are no large fluctuations in β during this set of trials. If this still occurs, it shows up as an effect on d' (Wagenaar, 1973). Although the assumption of a relatively stable criterion over time may be plausible, it is certainly not always valid. Thus, it may be doubtful in studies of vigilance and other conditions where motivational effects are thought to prevail (e.g., Warm and Jerison, 1984). Any short-term increases in the variance of β do not only remain undetected but are actually misinterpreted.

Both objections to error measures do not apply to forced choice reaction measures. Despite some uncertainties in actual measurement (e.g., Pachella, 1974), it is usually plausible to measure reaction time on a ratio scale, which has enormous advantages. It is not bedevilled by ceilings and permits a trial-by-trial analysis.

The analogue of criterion variability in signal detection measurement is the speed-accuracy problem in the measurement of reaction time. It is curious that as much as the problem of criterion variability has been neglected, the speed-accuracy issue has been emphasized, even to the point where time measures that do not consider the speed-accuracy trade-off have been out-lawed (Wickelgren, 1977). Only combined accuracy-latency functions would be permissible.

As I have argued elsewhere in greater detail (Sanders, 1980a), the speed-accuracy issue in choice reactions is twofold. First, there is the problem of random variation within a block of trials. Secondly, there is the issue of changes in speed-accuracy trade-off, and thus of reaction time, between blocks of trials as a result of an experimental variable. The last case is the most interesting, since it suggests a strategical change in speed-accuracy as the explanation of the effects of an independent variable. A closer scrutiny of such effects might be possible by actual measures of speed-accuracy functions, although I doubt whether the spontaneous effects of independent variables would invariably recur when, say, deadline methods are invoked to further specify the effects. But there are certainly studies in which speed-accuracy function have shed light on the effect of relative signal frequency on choice reactions (Harm and Lappin, 1973).

The situation is very different when considering within-block effects on a trial-by-trial basis. Except when they are the subject of special analysis (e.g., Laming, 1979), these effects are usually uninteresting; they cannot be approached through speed-accuracy analysis and they are perhaps optimally counteracted by practice that stresses low variance performance.

The possibilities of reaction time measurement with regard to linear stage analysis—and hence to the description of what could be some elementary modules in human performance—have been well documented, amended, attacked, and defended (e.g., Sanders, 1980b; Pieters, 1983). The debate is not yet over. Yet its value in assessing drug effects has been demonstrated in the work of Frowein (1981), which will be discussed in more detail by Debus and Börgens in this volume. It should be noted that more finegrained analyses are possible along the lines proposed by Laming (1979) and Rabbitt (1979)—perhaps in particular by studying the error-shock-effect—which should permit the study of strategic effects. Latency measures could be particularly useful in the chronometric sense of Posner (1978), which does not only refer to reaction time proper but also to time relations between electrophysiological measures, such as evoked potentials. The possibilities of measuring time relation in movements like handwriting and in high speed sequences of responses as in typing and piano playing carry the prospects of time measurement far beyond the discrete reaction time.

Yet our ultimate aim of approaching and predicting real life conditions should exclude any constraint on the method of measurement. The typical conditions, where error measures are commonly used—consider tracking, selective attention, working memory analyses, and dual task analysis—have provided an important set of suggestions with regard to the effects of the stressors (e.g., Welford, 1973; Hockey, 1979). As with more complex time measures, measures of error can also be elaborated to a greater degree of subtlety. Thus, one may think of a more finegrained motion analysis. Irrespective of time or error measures, there has always been the wish to get beyond what is directly given in reactions to stimuli. Although life is certainly more than a set of 'stranded episodes' (Shaffer, 1980) as studied in the laboratory, for the moment we will be limited to the types of experimental tasks that in fact consist of such stranded episodes (Sanders, 1984).

Conclusions

The questions remain: what type of tasks? Is the time ripe for a standardized battery? The answer may not be a straight yes or no. Rather one may think of a set of batteries to be validated in carefully chosen tasks or subtasks. The Fleishman battery certainly deserves closer scrutiny and comparison with more recent attempts. With regard to predictions of driving efficiency, Sanders (1986) suggested that a battery should contain a risk-taking test, preferably a simple compensatory tracking task with vague safety boundaries, a self-paced speed option, and a variable preview. The task should not normally provide the type of knowledge of results that adds to the attraction of current computer games. A combination of certain versions of this task with verbal comprehension tests could create a useful dual task setting in addition to determining single tracking performance. A third task could consist in a choice reaction test in which time uncertainty and stimulus quality are varied in order to include effects of suboptimal perceptual motor demands, In a multi-skill situation such as car driving, the tracking task would be the continuous element and the choice reaction the discrete element. The time is certainly ripe for a more concerted action towards composing and testing the usefulness of such batteries.

References

Baker WJ, Geist AM, and Fleishman EA (1967) *Effects of Cylert on Physiological and Psychomotor Performance Measures.* Tech. Rep. AIR-E-31. Washington D.C.: American Institute for Research.

Blaauw GJ (1977) Een geinstrumenteerde auto voor gedragsonderzoek op de weg. *Polytechnisch Tijdschrift* **32**, 491–5.

Borkenstein RF, Crother RF, Schumate RP, Ziel WB, and Zijlman R (1964) *The Role of Drinking Drivers in Traffic Accidents.* Department of Police Administration. Bloomington: Indiana University.

Elkin EH, Freedle RO, van Cott HP and Fleishman EA (1965) *Effects of Drugs on Human Performance: The Effects of Scopolamine on the Presentative Human Performance Tests.* Tech. Rep. AIR-E-25. Washington D.C.: American Institute for Research.

Fleishman EA (1982) Systems for describing human tasks. *Am. Psychol.* **37**, 821–34.

Fleishman EA (1985) *Human Task Taxonomies.* New York: Wiley.

Frowein HW (1981) Selective effects of barbiturate and amphetamine on information processing and response execution. *Acta Psychol.* **47**, 105–15.

Gaillard AWK and Varey CA (1979) Some effects of an ACTH. 4-9 analog on human performance. *Physiol. Behav.* **23**, 78–84.

Gopher D and Sanders AF (1984) S-oh-R: Oh Stages! Oh resources! In; Prinz W and Sanders AF (eds.) *Cognition and Motor Processes.* Heidelberg: Springer.

Harm OJ and Lappin JS (1973) Probability, compatibility, speed and accuracy. *J. Exp. Psychol.* **100**, 416–8.

Harris W (1977) Fatigue, circadian rhythm and truck accidents. In: Mackie RR (ed.) *Vigilance.* New York: Plenum Press.

Heuer H (1984) Motor learning as a process of structural construction and displacement. In: Prinz W and Sanders AF (eds.) *Cognition and Motor Processes.* Heidelberg: Springer.

Hindmarch I (1980) Psychomotor function and psychoactive drugs. *Br. J. Clin. Pharmacol.* **10**, 189–209.

Hockey GRJ (1979) Stress and the cognitive components of skilled performance. In: Hamilton V and Warburton DM (eds.) *Human Stress and Cognition.* New York: Wiley.

Laming D (1979) Choice reaction performance following an error. *Acta Psychologica* **43**, 199–224.

Näätänen R, Simpson M and Leveless NE (1982) Stimulus deviance and evoked potentials. *Biol. Psychol.* **14**, 53–98.

Neisser U (1976) *Cognition and Reality.* San Francisco: Freeman.

O'Hanlon J and de Gier J (eds.) (1986) *Drugs and Driving.* London: Taylor Francis.

O'Hanlon J, Haak TW, Blaauw GJ and Riemersma JBJ. (1982) Diazepam impairs lateral position control in highway driving. *Science,* **217**, 79–81.

Pachella RG (1974) The interpretation of reaction time in information processing. In Kautowitz B (ed.) *Tutorials in performance and cognition* New Jersey: Erlbaum.

Pieters JPM (1983) Sternberg's additive factor method and underlying psychological processes: some theoretical considerations. *Psychol. Bull.* **93**, 411–26.

Posner MI (1978) *Chronometric Explorations of Mind.* Hillsdale NJ.: Erlbaum.

Rabbitt PMA (1979) Current paradigms and models in human information processing. In: Hamilton W and Warburton DM (eds.) *Human Stress and Cognition.* New York: Wiley.

Riemersma JBJ, Sanders AF, Wildervanck C and Gaillard AWK (1977) Performance decrement during prolonged night driving. In: Mackie RR (ed.) *Vigilance.* New York: Plenum Press.

Sanders AF (1976) Experimental methods in human engineering. In: Kraiss KF and Moraal J (eds.) *Introduction to Human Engineering.* TÜV Rheinland: Verlag.

Sanders AF (1980a) Some effects of instructed muscle tension on choice reaction time and movement time. In: Nickerson RS (ed.) *Attention and Performance 8.* Hillsdale, New Jersey: Erlbaum.

Sanders AF (1980b) Stage analysis of reaction processes. In: Stelmach GE and Requin I (eds.) *Tutorials in Motor Behaviour.,* Amsterdam: North Holland.

Sanders AF (1983) Towards a model of stress and human performance. *Acta Psychol.* **53**, 61–97.

Sanders AF (1984) Ten symposia on attention and performance: Some issues and trends. In: Bouma H and Bouwhuis D (eds.) *Attention and Performance 10.* Hillsdale, New Jersey: Erlbaum.

Sanders AF (1986) Drugs, driving and the measurement of performance. In: O'Hanlon JF and de Gier J (eds.) *Drugs and Driving.* London: Taylor Francis.

Shaffer LH (1973) Latency mechanisms in transcription. In: Kornblum S (ed.) *Attention and Performance 4.* London: Academic Press.

Shaffer LH (1975) Multiple attention in continuous verbal tasks. In: Rabbitt PMA and Dornic S (eds.) *Attention and Performance 5.* London: Academic Press.

Shaffer LH (1980) Book review. *Q. J. Exp. Psychol.* **32**, 174–6.

Shaffer LH (1981) Performances of Chopin, Bach, and Bartok: Studies in motor-programming. *Cognitive Psychol.* **13**, 326–76.

Shingledecker CA (1984) A taskbattery for applied human performance assessment research. *AFAMRL-TR.* 84–071. Wright Patterson AFB.

Theologus GC, Wheaton GR and Fleishman EA (1974) Effects of intermittent, moderate intensity noise-stress on human performance., *J. Appl. Psychol.* **59**, 539–47.

Truyens, CL and Schuffel H (1978) Ergonomisch onderzoek 'Open Hartelkanaal': Validering van de simulatie von duvaart in het Hartelgebied. Rapport IZF-1978-C-6.

Wagenaar WA (1973) The effect of fluctuations *of vcopone criterion* and sensitivity in a signal detection experiment. *Psychologische Forschung.*

Warm JS and Jerison HJ (1984) The psychophysics of vigilance. In: Warm JS (ed.) *Sustained Attention in Human Performance.* New York: Wiley.

Welford AT (1973) Stress and human performance. *Ergonomics* **16**, 567–80.

Wickens CD (1984) Processing resources in attention. In Parasuraman R and Davies DR (eds.) *Varieties of Attention*. New York: Academic Press.

Wicklegren WA (1977) Speed-accuracy trade off and information processing dynamics. *Acta Psychol.* **41**, 67–85.

Psychopharmacology and Reaction Time
Edited by I. Hindmarch, B. Aufdembrinke and H. Ott
© 1988 John Wiley & Sons Ltd

11

Localization in the Stimulus- and Response-contingent Brain Activity in a Forced-choice Detection Task

K. Kranda, P Cheruy, M. Jobert and H. Ott

Schering Research Laboratories, Berlin/Bergkamen, FRG

Introduction

In this chapter we address the question of how to measure several psycho-physical, behavioural, and electrophysiological parameters simultaneously and how various types of data processing can increase the information content gained from such an experiment. It is not our intention at this stage to offer well-meant advice to psychopharmacologists on the suitability or unsuitability of various tests. The main thrust of this investigation is to explore different routes towards an economical localization and identification of various neural processes of the human brain. The methodology described here has not been developed exclusively for psychotropic drug testing but also as a general tool for investigating brain function.

The measurement of reaction times (RTs) is a simple way of assessing the effects of psychotropic drugs on performance. Indeed, many drugs do affect RTs to sensory stimulation, but this observation is neither particularly surprising in itself nor does it provide much insight into the nature of drug action on the central nervous system (CNS). Moreover, it does not give much useful information about the mechanisms of signal processing, primarily because it is not easy to separate the neural processes participating in, say, detection from RTs. RT measurement cannot even easily separate direct effects on given neural structures from indirect ones, such as pupilary diameter, fixation, accommodation, or corneal irritation. The contribution of such indirect effects to RTs either cannot be directly assessed or requires the application of other techniques. Likewise, the role of attention and motivation in RT measurements under drugs cannot easily be assessed.

If RTs alone cannot provide much insight into the mechanisms of drug action, one may have to consider combining measures with some other methods of applying additional controls to minimize the influence of undesirable variables. The simultaneous recording of RTs and electrical potentials from the human scalp seems at present the most convenient technique, since it can provide an electrophysiological correlate of a motor response to a given sensory stimulus.

The electrical activity recorded from the brain can be averaged and synchronized in time either with the onset of the stimulus (stimulus-contingent averaging) or with the start of the subject's response (response-contingent averaging). In our studies both types of averaging were performed on the same set of results. Response-contingent averaging was included to reveal decision processes in a forced-choice task which led to the formulation of the response. This was done to provide additional information about the nature of RTs, since most experiments have almost exclusively used stimulus-contingent averaging (Donchin, 1984).

The electrophysiological correlates of the responses in a detection task were identified by applying the Laplacean operator and response-contingent averaging, which was directly synchronized with the subject's response. The Laplacean derivation allowed the spatial separation of the various electrophysiological components.

Furthermore, the content of individual sweeps was examined by a cross-correlation procedure. This technique allows a statistical evaluation of the similarity between the average (a template) and an individual sweep. However, neither this technique nor various forms of time-varying filtering (De Weerd and Kap, 1981; Yu and McGillem, 1983) can easily answer the fundamental problem of signal stationarity or amplitude variability. This is principally because of the poor signal-to-noise ratio of the electrophysiological signals and the overlap between the noise and signal spectra. Thus the presence, the absence, or the latency of a signal can only be considered in probabilistic terms.

Methods

Stimuli

A sine-wave grating of 6 c/deg appeared for 50 msec in the subject's right visual field just above or below a fixation point at the centre of a visual display subtending $4°$ of visual angle. The grating patterns subtending $1°$ of visual field were presented in a pseudorandom order which allowed an equal number of presentations to both locations. The stimuli were generated by modulating the Z-axis of a Tektronix CRT display. A window generator allowed the presentation of a spatially discrete pattern anywhere on the screen while maintaining the average luminance constant. The contrast and spatial frequency of the gratings were set externally by a PDP 11/23 through two analogue outputs of an A/D converter. In two separate sessions, the contrast of the grating (defined according to the Michelson formula as $C = L_{max} - L_{min}/L_{max} + L_{min}$, where L_{max} and L_{min} are the luminance maxima and minima of the screen) was set either to 0.25 (1 log unit above threshold) or to its threshold value of 0.025 at which the subject was able to make a correct response in a forced-choice task (up or down) with 75% accuracy. The contrast of the gratings was calibrated with a Pin 10 photocell (UDT) attached to an optical assembly such that it was possible to focus the phosphor layer (P 31) of the CRT with a microscope lens ($\times 10$). The diameter of the spot measured on the surface of the screen was 0.1 mm. The grating of the screen was made to drift slowly while the output of the photocell, which was synchronized with phase of the drift, was sampled at 256 Hz by the computer with one channel of an A/D converter. Averaging of 32 sweeps reduced noise and improved the accuracy of the data. The contrast of the grating was computed automatically. The recorded waveform was analyzed with a FFT routine in order to assure spectral purity of the pattern. The average luminance of the screen, which was kept constant throughout the experiments, was set to 80 cd/m^2, at which there was no distortion of the sinewave pattern. The average luminance of the screen run at the frame rate of 100 Hz was determined by integrating the photocell output with an electronic filter whose corner frequencies were set to DC and 35 Hz ($-$ 8 dB) in order to approximate the temporal properties of the visual system.

Recording

The evoked potentials were recorded with 14 channels of a Nihon Koden EEG system. The filter characteristic and the sensitivity of all the channels were calibrated by applying attenuated outputs of a function generator to the amplifiers. The sensitivity of all the channels was matched to within 2%; the corner frequencies of the filters (0.7–35 Hz) were matched to within 5%. The recording was unipolar, referenced to linked ears, and grounded to an electrode on the subject's forehead. The electrode array was triangular in order to maximize the ratio of central electrodes to the total. This arrangement (see Figure 1) was used to calculate Laplacean derivations (Nunez, 1981; Mackay, 1983, 1984). The six central electrodes were placed along the vertical midline and were spaced regularly at 5% of the nasion–inion distance of 36 cm. The remaining six electrodes were positioned along the midline equidistant (18 mm) from their counterparts. The impedance of all the electrodes was matched at about 2 kΩ. The electric signals were amplified and digitalized (12 bit A/D) at 256 points per second. The recording period, i.e., a single sweep, lasted 1 sec.

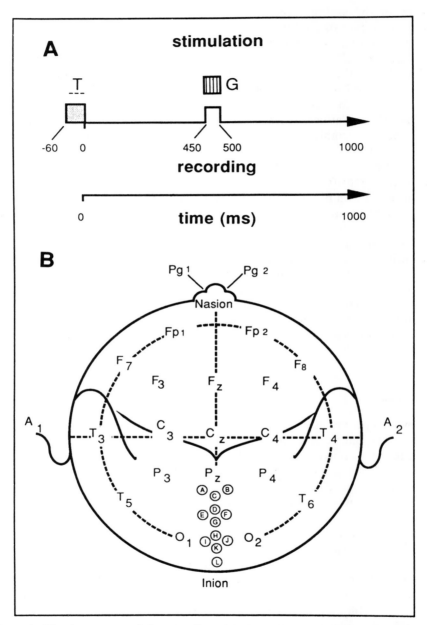

Figure 1. The time course of the recording and stimulating procedures. T signifies the period within which a tone indicated that the grating onset G was imminent. The diagram below illustrates the position of a spatial array of 12 electrodes A to L.

Procedure

A warning tone (a short bleep) was sounded at random intervals 60, 50, 40, 30, 20, and 10 msec before or at the beginning of a recording period of 1000 msec. This was done to avoid synchronization of the tone with the visual signal. The grating appeared for 50 msec 450 msec after the beginning of the sweep (see Figure 1). The intertrial interval was 3 sec. The left-handed subject fixated the centre of the screen and had to respond as fast as possible (within 500 msec of stimulus onset) to the spatial location of the stimulus, i.e., above or below the fixation point, with the appropriate thumb (left for up and right for down).

Two averaging epochs of 500 msec were used. The first began with the onset of the grating and ended 500 msec later (stimulus-contingent averaging). The second began 500 msec before each response and terminated at the instance of the response (response-contingent averaging), i.e., counting back in time from the point of the response. The electrophysiological signal for the four possible response categories, i.e. (a) above-correct, (b) above-incorrect, (c) below-correct, and (d) below-incorrect were averaged separately. The subject's responses, that is the reaction times for each of the four conditions, were also processed separately. The reaction times, integrated within 25 msec bins, were displayed as frequency of response histograms.

Single treatment and analysis

The signal-to-noise ratio was increased using two filtering procedures:

1. Adaptive filtering, whereby individual sweeps were evaluated in terms of similarity to the average (i.e., a cross-correlation of the template with the individual sweeps; see Woody, 1967, for a similar procedure). The quartile of the sweep that was least similar to the template was taken out, and a new average was computed.
2. Time-varying filtering (see De Weerd and Kap, 1981) utilizing a bank of proportional bandwidth filters.

Results

The response-contingent EPs measured at contrasts of 0.25 and 0.025, i.e., at threshold, arbitrarily defined as the contrast giving 75% correct response in a forced-choice task, are shown in Figure 2 (panels A and B). The actual proportion of the correct responses at 0.025 contrast (an average of 16 blocks of 64 presentations each) was 76% and thus very close the ideal value. The contrast of 0.025 was also set by the subject (a method of adjustment) as her threshold value. The requirement of a rapid response in the forced-choice task thus had no noticeable effect on the proportion of correct responses.

Only results for electrode sites along the midline are shown here. In panel A of Figure 2, three components can be identified: (a) A negativity with a maximum at about 160 msec (lower visual field) or about 180 msec (upper visual field). (b) A minor negativity at about 250 msec which is more prominent for the lower visual field presentations at suprathreshold levels. This component is more prominent for threshold presentation in panel B. (c) A

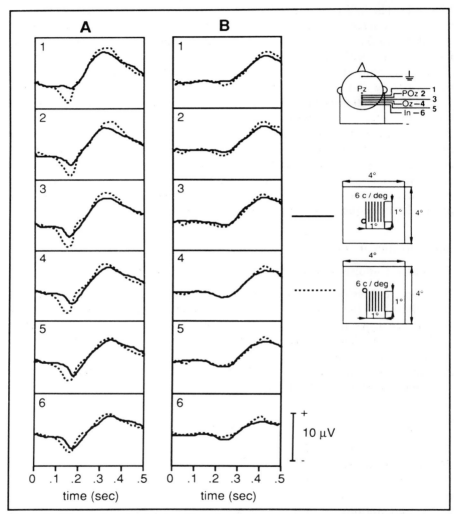

Figure 2. The t.v.f and adaptive filtered stimulus-contingent averages of 512 sweeps for detection of 6 c/deg gratings of 0.25(A) and 0.025 threshold (B) contrast. The numbers of the individual traces correspond to electrode locations along the midline (see the inset). The recording was unipolar and referenced to the linked ears. The averages are for correct responses only (76% of the total at threshold).

positivity at about 330 msec. A similar positivity is evident in the threshold condition in panel B but with a latency of about 415 msec. Yet whether the two components are related cannot easily be decided by visual inspection alone.

The different rates of grating detectability, however, complicate the issue. For gratings whose contrast was 10 times the threshold value, the error rate—presumably reflecting confusion unrelated to stimulus perception when the subject pressed the wrong button—was well below 1% of the total responses (512 left and 512 right).

At threshold, however, detectability was 76%, but we were unable to establish what proportion of the responses was purely due to chance. Let us assume for the sake of simplicity that the chance level was about 50% and that only about 25% of the 512 sweeps actually contained the signal. Because of the proportion of correct responses due to chance, one might expect the signal-to-noise ratio to be halved (i.e., a square root of 4) and the amplitude of the positive wave to be about half that in panel B. As this is not the case, one can consider two *ad hoc* explanations:

1. The proportion of correct responses attributed to chance is much less than 50%.
2. The late positive component in panel A is a compound wave containing a late visual component that is contrast dependent and another positive wave corresponding to the active participation in the task (cf. Figure 6 of Parry *et al.*, chapter 13, this volume). Thus if the contrast-dependent component disappeared at threshold, the other component would still be present and manifest itself as the late wave at 415 msec.

Assuming that the second option is more plausible because of the relatively small proportion of very short responses (see Figure 9), then the problem that has still to be resolved is to what extent this wave depends on the response mode, i.e., correct or incorrect. In Figure 3 the late components generated during incorrect responses are not easily identifiable. (Note that only results for the inferior right quadrant are shown since those for the superior field are essentially identical.) This may at first seem to be a paradox, since the late component is contrast independent but at the same time depends on the subject's capacity to correctly identify the stimulus. Perhaps this component depends on the capacity to detect the stimulus in just two modes, seen or not seen, which is essentially a decision process.

In order to elucidate some of the decision processes leading to the formulation of the response, i.e., seen or not seen, we employed a response-contingent averaging technique, whereby the end of each epoch was synchronized with the onset of the subject's response. The waveforms in Figure 4A are relatively independent of the retinal location of the stimuli. The curves in panel B are identical in terms of stimulus location and the hand used to effect the response. This latter point implies that if there is a ERP lateralization

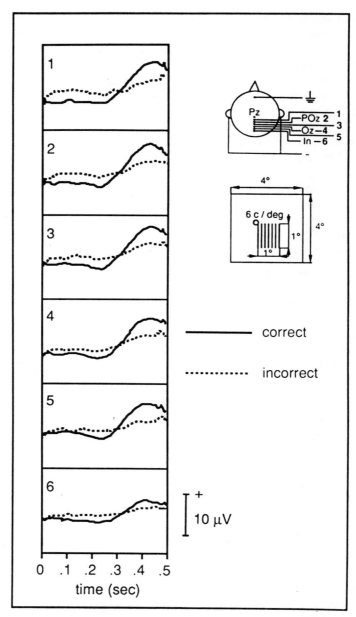

Figure 3. A comparison of unipolar recordings for correct (solid curves) and incorrect (dashed curves) responses to the 6 c/deg grating at threshold. The proportions of correct and incorrect responses were 76% and 24% respectively.

depending on the dexterity of the response, it is not manifested in these recordings from the occipital and parietal regions. Note also that the difference between curves for inferior and superior field presentation tends to disappear at threshold for both stimulus- (Figure 2) and response-contingent averaging (Figure 4).

Although the curves in panels A and B should be equivalent inasmuch as

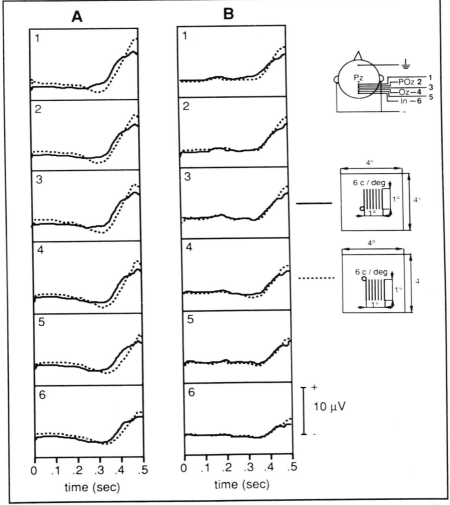

Figure 4. Response-contingent averaging of EPs, 500 msec prior to the response (the response occurred here at 0.5 sec). The recording was unipolar. The two panels correspond to correct detection responses to gratings above (A) and at threshold (B).

they should represent the same decision process leading to a correct response, they are not identical. The significance of the slightly different amplitude is impossible to assess, but at threshold the decision process possibly corresponding to the negativity is somewhat faster (about 50 msec).

The amplitudes of all the components gradually increase with distance from the inion, indicating that the maximum of these curves is more central and thus outside of the electrode array.

If there is relatively good correspondence between curves for correct responses, i.e., where the location of the grating has been identified correctly (the proportion of correct responses due to chance is not considered here as it cannot easily be assessed; the only indicators are the proportions of very short responses below 200 msec in Figure 9), a comparison can be made with ERPs for incorrect responses, i.e., when the subject presumably could not detect the stimulus. This is shown in Figure 5, where at threshold contrast the proportion of incorrect responses was 24% of the total. The picture here is very different from that seen in Figure 4: the only discernible negativity has an extremely short latency at about 50 msec and is more prominent for presentations to the superior hemifield. The gradual increase of its amplitude with increasing proximity to the central brain region (from being almost totally absent at the inion) and the short latency suggest that this component corresponds to a purely motor response which has its peak activity outside of the electrode array used in this experiment.

The results of the unipolar recording cannot provide sufficiently accurate information about the origin of the various components. For instance, ERPs from unipolar recordings contain components generated outside of the electrode array and components originating in deep (subcortical) regions of the brain. In order to facilitate an analysis of the ERP components, we computed Laplacean derivations for the electrodes along the midline (see Figure 5). In contrast to the small number of ERP waves in Figure 2, whose amplitude of the late components increases with distance from the inion, the Laplacean derivations for five locations along the midline in Figure 6 show a surprisingly large number of various components, but only for the suprathreshold condition (see panel A). None of the components has a latency longer than 300 msec, where unipolar waves show their maxima (see Figure 2). The early components tend to differ for presentation to the upper and lower visual fields. At locations 2 and 4, two early components at about 90 msec and 120 msec are apparent, but only for the lower visual field presentation. The later components, especially the negativity at about 220 msec and the positivity at 270 msec, show a much greater spatial distribution and seem less dependent on the retinal position of the gratings. The dual polarity reversal indicates the possible multiplicity of the sources, or the presence of a sulcus separating one neural structure. At threshold (see panel B) no components can be clearly recognized. Note that the scale in B is different since the curves were flat when

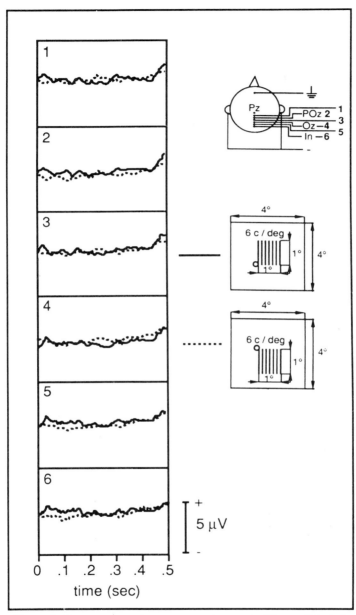

Figure 5. Response-contingent averaging as in Figure 7 but for incorrect responses.

plotted on an identical scale. The inability to identify any of the components present in panel A suggests a contrast-specific nature of the Laplacean derivations shown in panel A. The apparent contrast nonspecificity of the curves from unipolar recordings suggests that their origin is outside of the electrode array. The Laplacean curves for the incorrect responses were also flat and are not shown here.

The Laplacean derivations of response-contingent averaging (see Figure 7) for grating detection above threshold show some unexpected differences between superior and inferior hemifield presentations. At threshold, no Laplacean EP components for correct or incorrect responses could be identified. The spatial distribution of these components seems to obey a similar

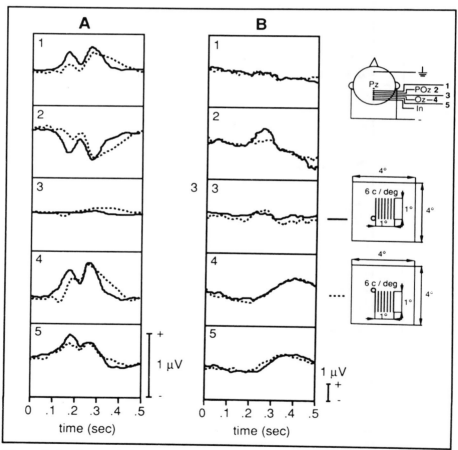

Figure 6. Laplacean derivations for detection of gratings of 25% (A) and 2.5% (B) contrast.

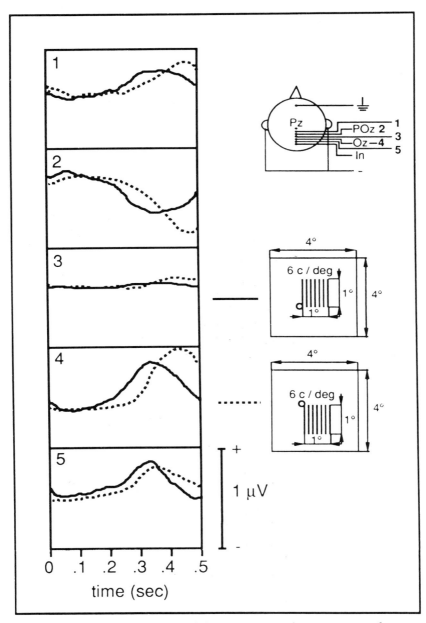

Figure 7. Laplacean derivatives of the response-continent averages of correct responses to gratings above threshold.

pattern (symmetry around electrode number three positioned 18 mm above POz) to that observed for stimulus-contingent averaging (see Figure 6).

Finally, we present reaction time histograms of responses to the gratings. We decided to present the RTs as histograms rather than as grand averages with standard deviations since the former convey more information about the response distributions (see Tolhurst, 1975; Kranda, 1983). The response histograms for suprathreshold gratings are shown in Figure 8. The RTs were integrated here within bins of 25 msec each. The vertical dashed lines indicate the mean RTs for each condition.

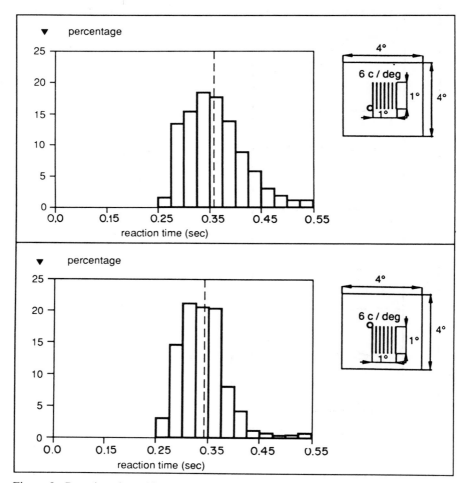

Figure 8. Reaction-time histograms for suprathreshold gratings presented above (upper distribution) and below (lower distribution) the fixation point. The vertical dashed lines indicate the means. The responses were integrated within 25 msec bins.

The broader distribution of the RTs to gratings presented to the superior hemifield reflects the subject's greater response uncertainty. The average RTs to gratings located in the inferior hemifield are also shorter by about 20 msec (289 msec compared with 311 msec). Figures 9 and 10 represent RT distributions at threshold for correct and incorrect responses, shown separately for the two hemifield presentations. The distributions in Figure 9 are even broader than in Figure 8, corresponding to the great response uncertainty at threshold and also reflecting a small number of correct responses due to chance. Note the very flat histogram for incorrect responses to gratings presented to the superior

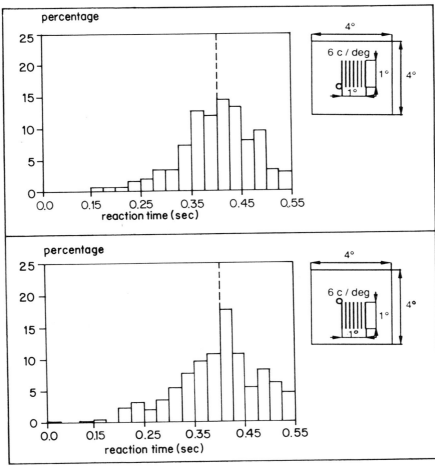

Figure 9. Reaction-time histograms for correct responses to gratings at threshold.

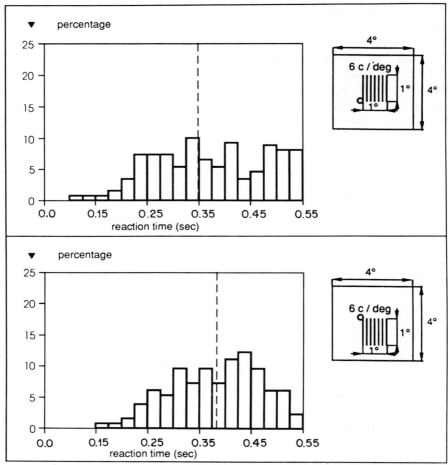

Figure 10. Reaction-time histograms for incorrect responses to gratings at threshold.

hemifield, indicating the random nature of the response even though the subject heard a warning tone 510–450 msec before the onset of the grating. The average RTs for incorrect responses also tend to be shorter (322 msec and 332 msec) than their counterparts for the correct responses (347 msec and 349 msec).

Discussion

The major item of information gained in this study was the demonstration that it is feasible to partially separate various contributions of the neural centres to the late complex waves such as P300.

When trying to find a correspondence between the latency of, say, a P300 wave and RTs, we are faced with the difficulty of establishing to what extent it can be considered a unitary wave. The picture that emerges from unipolar recordings casts some doubt on the unitary nature of the late waves. The late positivity (P300) seems to be composed of several components with different origins. For instance, at suprathreshold the P300 components recorded at locations near Pz (see Figure 2) display some elements of retinotopicity, i.e., they differ for upper and lower field presentations. This retinotopic component disappears at threshold, suggesting that the sensory components of P300 are too small to be apparent at threshold. Thus the P300 wave that is composite contains sensory components which can be separated. These components obey retinotopic organization and are contrast dependent. Yet one of the sensory components is not an off response to the stimulus, because the subject does not have any off response to 6 c/deg gratings. Moreover, the P300 amplitudes for detecting gratings at threshold are no greater than their counterparts measured at 10 times the threshold contrast, even though one might expect this on the basis of a Donchin hypothesis of proportionality between the probability of an appearance and an amplitude. Although the grating is presented every time, at threshold the subjective appearance is below 75%, since some of the correct responses are due to chance. The amplitude of the late components seems not to be influenced by the probability of a subjective appearance (corresponding to detection).

If P300 in general had the curious facility of being present even in the absence of a stimulus (see Ruchkin and Sutton, 1978) and assuming that such a condition is equivalent to not seeing the stimulus—and would lead to an incorrect response in a forced-choice task—it should not differ much for correct and incorrect responses. Yet the absence of any identifiable P300 component (see Figure 3) in the comparison of correct and incorrect responses fails to confirm such a hypothesis and indicates that the components here may have different origins than those reported elsewhere. It is unclear to what extent the presence of P300 depends on the presence of the stimulus or on the mode of response, i.e., correct versus incorrect (cf. also figure of McGlone *et al.* in this volume, which shows a comparison of P300 waves for correct and incorrect responses in a discrimination task).

Uncertainty concerning the estimation of ERP latencies

Note also the rather random distribution of RTs for incorrect responses in Figure 10 and compare these with results for correct responses in Figure 9. One could argue, however, that the latency of the individual responses can be correlated with the latencies of the appropriate waveforms. Yet this procedure may not yield the desired effect because of the theoretical limitations of identifying a waveform in noise without the appropriate template (a P300 from another set of experiments could be employed, but only at the cost of accuracy). Moreover, the assumption that it is possible to identify and localize a signal in note violates Heisenberg's principle of indeterminacy. Gabor (1946) applied this principle in his communication theory, which states that one cannot simultaneously localize a signal within an infinitely narrow time interval and frequency band.

Response-contingent averaging

It would appear that the average RTs to gratings at threshold are not much longer than those measured at 10 times their contrast. This is primarily because some of the correct responses were due to chance. This may partially explain why the latency of the P300 roughly corresponds to the average RTs above threshold but is much longer at threshold. But the latencies of the late waves are in any case too long to reflect the decision processes leading to the response. This is a paradox, since the components convey some information about detection (cf. Figure 3) for correct and incorrect responses). Yet the actual decision process synchronized with the response must occur earlier. This was revealed by response-contingent averaging and appeared as a major negativity preceding the response by about 180 msec above threshold, and by about 150 msec at threshold. This negativity probably represents a decision process rather than a formulation of the response as such, since no equivalent wave could be identified for ERPs preceding the incorrect responses.

Laplacean derivations

In order to aid the identification of the late waves (e.g., P300) from unipolar recordings, we computed Laplacean derivations for grating detection above and at threshold (see Figure 6). The Laplacean derivatives for gratings at threshold (panel B) are not discernible (note the scale), suggesting a different origin from those for suprathreshold gratings (see panel A). The two P300 waves in Figure 2 are thus rather different from each other although superficially they may appear similar. The P300 wave recorded in the suprathreshold condition contains sensory elements (cf. Figure 6A), whereas the P300 recorded at threshold has origins outside of the electrode array. The dual polarity reversal observed between recording locations just above the inion and just short of the Pz (see Figure 6A) suggest a multiple origin of the derived components.

The Laplacean derivation for response-contingent averaging above threshold revealed several components which seem to depend on the position of the grating in the visual field. These components are localized above the visual and associative areas and cannot correspond to the dexterity of the response left versus right since they cannot be identified in the threshold condition.

Conclusion

In this study the application of the Laplacean operator demonstrated that it is possible to separate and localize brain activity better than the traditional unipolar recordings. The combination of the stimulus- and response-contingent allows a comparison of detection and decision processes.

References

De Weerd JPC and Kap JI (1981) A posteriori time varying filtering of averaged evoked potentials. Mathematical and computational aspect *Biol. Cybern.* **41**, 223–34.

Donchin E (1984) *Cognitive Psychology*, Hillsdale, New Jersey:

Gabor D (1946) Theory of communication. *IEEE* **93**, 429–57.

Kranda K (1983) Analysis of reaction times to coloured stimuli. *Ophthalmic Physiol. Opt.* **3**, 223–31.

Mackay DM (1983) On-line source-density computation with a minimum of electrodes. *Electroencephalogr. Clin. Neurophysiol.* **57**, 233–7.

Mackay DM (1984) Source density analysis of scalp potentials during evaluated action. I. coronal distribution. *Exp. Brain. Res.* **54**, 73–85.

Nunez PL (1981) *Electric Fields of the Brain*. Oxford: Oxford University Press.

Ruchkin DS and Sutton S (1978) Equivocation and P300 amplitude. In: Ott O (ed.) *Multidisciplinary Perspectives in Event-Related Potential Research*. EPA 600/9-77-043. Washington, DC: GPO

Tolhurst DJ (1975) Reaction times in the detection of gratings by human observers. *Vision Res.* **15**, 1143–9.

Woody CD (1967) Characterisation of an adaptive filter for the analysis of variable latency neuroelectric signals. *Med. Biol. Eng.* **4**, 539–53.

Yu K-B and McGillem CD (1983) Optimum filters for estimating evoked potentials waveforms. *IEEE Trans. Biomed. Eng.* **30**, 730–7.

Psychopharmacology and Reaction Time
Edited by I. Hindmarch, B. Aufdembrinke and H. Ott
© 1988 John Wiley & Sons Ltd

12

Post-ingestion Effects of Benzodiazepines on Evoked Potentials and Reaction Times in Discrimination Tasks

F. P. McGlone[1], *J. J. Kulikowski*[1], *K. Kranda*[2], *and H. Ott*[2]

[1]*Visual Sciences Laboratory, University of Manchester Institute of Science and Technology, Manchester, UK*
[2]*Schering Research Laboratories, Berlin/Bergkamen, FRG*

Introduction

The processes involved in the discrimination of briefly flashed amoeboid shapes tend to evoke scalp potentials whose two late waves (cf. Ciesielski, 1982) resemble the N200 and P300 waves widely reported elsewhere (see for instance Donchin, 1984). As the amoeboid shapes have no verbal connotation and hardly differ in physical parameters such as contrast, luminance or hue, some higher form of processing (i.e., with elements of cognition) is needed for their discrimination. This feature was considered desirable for testing some subtle effects of long-acting drugs one day after ingestion (cf. Kulikowski *et al.*, 1984). The above study not only demonstrated the feasibility of providing an electrophysiological index of a drug action during a discrimination task, but also provided the most sensitive indicator (a 30% reduction of amplitude) in a group of several tests.

The purpose of the present study is twofold. First, to examine to what extent the discrimination of amoeboid shapes is a unique way of giving a good index of drug action or whether some other discrimination tasks utilizing different types of stimulation are just as effective, if not more so. This investigation also serves partially as a control for previous studies (Kulikowski *et al.*, 1984) by testing alternative stimulus parameters. We included length discrimination of vertical lines, which has been reported to correlate with intelligence (Mackintosh, 1981). The second aim was to assess closely the effects of acute drug administration on reaction times (RTs) and evoked potentials (EPs).

Methods

Stimuli

The same amoeboid shapes were used as described by Ciesielski (1982) and Ciesielski *et al.* (1983), except that in this study they were generated on a television monitor (Grundig F3015) and presented for 60 msec. The shapes appeared paracentrally (in this case $3° 45'$) to the left or right of the fixation point at the centre of the display. In one control experiment the shapes were presented to the centre of the display. As the presentations were randomized, the subject was forced to fixate the central point in order to optimize the number of correct responses. The sequence of pairs with same or different shapes was also randomized in order to prevent responses on the basis of expectancy. Each block of 32 presentations contained 16 pairs of the same and 16 pairs of different shapes.

The second kind of stimuli were pairs of vertical lines of either equal or different lengths. The mean length corresponded to $1°$ of the visual angle. The different lines deviated by 20% of this mean value. In the preliminary stage of this study three types of presentation were examined: parallel lines presented unilaterally, bilaterally presented lines, and vertically displaced lines (gap of $30'$) presented unilaterally. This last mode was adopted in the main study because it was comparable to that used for amoeboid shapes. The subject fixated the centre of the display and had to respond to each presentation by flopping two switches simultaneously with both hands, indicating whether the two shapes or lines in a pair were same or different. The subject's RTs to the mere appearance of the stimuli (i.e. detection RTs) were also measured.

Recording techniques

The arrangement was essentially the same as described by Kulikowski *et al.* (1984) except for the locations of the recording electrodes. These were positioned along the vertical midline at Oz, Pz, and in the drug study at Cz. This time, however, a Medelec sensor recording system was used. The electrophysiological signals were averaged on line, but some were also recorded on a FM tape recorder for subsequent selective averaging of individual sweeps carried out off-line.

Subjects

The subjects were healthy males with normal visual acuity (before or after correction). Four males participated in the nondrug (control) part of the study, and eight subjects were also tested during the recruitment procedure for the drug study. Two of these (J.K. and B.M., aged 47 and 34 years) were 'well-calibrated' subjects, i.e., subjects for whom a large collection of results is available for comparison.

Three subjects took part in the drug study; their previous experimental experience was limited to the preliminary testing that was part of the subject selection procedure. These subjects were neither aware of the purpose of the experiment nor of the nature (drug or placebo) of the administered substance. Each substance administration was separated by a one-week washout period.

Results

Effects of central and paracentral stimulus presentation on VEPs

This investigation formed part of the control experiments carried out on four subjects, but only the results of J.K. and B.M. are presented here. We have mentioned earlier (Kulikowski *et al.*, 1984) that paracentral presentation is advantageous for testing left-right asymmetries of the brain (cortex). There is, however, an additional advantage: paracentral presentation minimizes the early VEP components of sensory origin that may clash or coincide with waves generated during a discrimination (cognitive) task. This point is illustrated in Figure 1, which shows an experiment in which vertically displaced amoeboid shapes were presented either at fixation point or 3.75° to the left or right of this.

Passive viewing of paracentrally presented shapes elicited very small and unclear VEPs (see Figure 1 bottom left). This presumably reflects the substantial magnification of the central foveal representation in the visual cortex. In such cases any involvement in a task produces a potential, a prominent feature of which is a positive wave that peaks between 200 and 300 msec. This is illustrated in Figure 1 (mid-left) which depicts the situation when the subject was asked to count the presentations. This potential, however, is still small; a substantial increase was achieved only when the subject was asked to differentiate between same or different shapes (Figure 1, top left). Note that the most prominent complex is the well-documented negative (N200) and positive (P300) complex (for a review see Hillyard and Kutas, 1983).

The passive observation of centrally presented shapes produces VEPs with small early negative-positive components (times to peak of about 90–100 msec) and prominent late negative (130 msec) and positive (P200) waves. In subject J.K. (Figure 1) the waveforms have different latencies at the parietal Pz site. When the subject was asked to count presentations, the VEPs at Oz did not change from those for passive viewing, but the VEPs recorded at Pz showed a shift of the positive peak as if a P300 component had been added. In the discrimination task, the purely visual components are clearly superimposed on the cognitive components, and the resulting waveform has a smaller

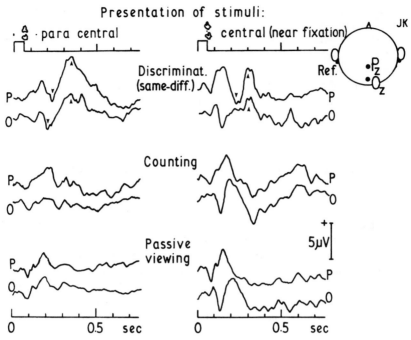

Figure 1. Demonstration of advantages of paracentral presentations (left column) over central presentations of the pairs of shapes (right column). Central presentations elicit stronger 'purely visual' VEPs (when the subject is passive) which then subtract from the 'cognitive' components when the subject is asked to discriminate 'same' and 'different' shapes (top row). Note the intermediate size of the VEPs when the subject is asked to count presentations (middle row).

amplitude than after paracentral presentation. The detection of gratings has also shown composite waves of added sensory and task-contingent components when the subject responds to the presentation (cf. Kranda *et al.* in this volume). It would appear that paracentral presentations permit a better separation of unilaterally recorded sensory and cognitive components than do central presentations. Laplacean derivation, however, allows a still better separation of waveforms even generated by centrally presented stimuli.

Effects of prolonged repetitive stimulation (habituation)

Figure 2 shows the effects of repetitive presentation (64 trials). Subject J.K. showed a substantial reduction of cognitive components in the course of the four experimental sessions (each of 16 repetitions). The late positive wave was largest at the beginning of the experiment but gradually diminished in the

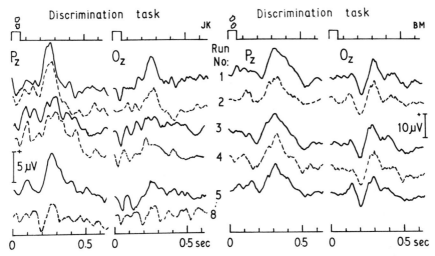

Figure 2. Effect of habituation on the 'cognitive' VEP components. In one paradigm the subject was presented with the same task (shape discrimination as in Figure 1) repeatedly four times (see records 1–4, left). Subsequently he was given a 10 minute break and the VEP magnitude recovered slightly (record 5, left) but then in the subsequent three sessions it was gradually reduced (see record 8, left). In the other paradigm (right column) the subject was allowed a break after each session and the VEP amplitude could be kept on a constant level.

course of four sessions. A-10 minute break after the fourth session partially restored the amplitude size (see trace 5), but it diminished again during the next three sessions.

In order to maintain the EP (P300) at a constant level and thus prevent habituation, subject B.M. (right panel) was allowed a break after each session, and the boredom of performing the task was relieved by rewarding him for each correct discrimination of the stimulus (same or different).

On the nature of cognitive EPs

Figure 3 shows separately averaged waveforms for correct and false judgements (optimal ratio 2:1 correct to false, i.e., about two thirds of the responses were correct). The results are for a matched number of correct and false responses; since the number of correct responses was twice that of false judgements, evoked potentials for every other correct judgement and all potentials for the false were averaged. Note that the last waves (dotted) for B.M. have only 14 repetitons since the subject made too few false judgements. It apears that for both subjects the waves generated by false judgements were only slightly broader than the waves elicited by correct judgments.

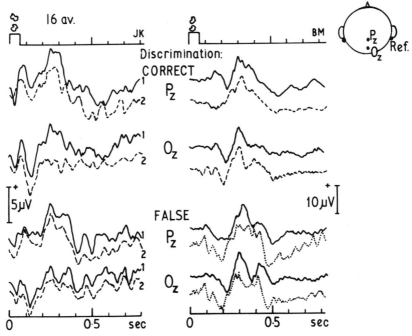

Figure 3. A comparison of EP waveforms for correct and incorrect responses to amoeboid figures for two subjects J.K. and B.M. The two traces in each condition (1 and 2) represent results of two separate runs. Sixteen trials were averaged in each case except for one condition, subject B. M. (dotted lines) who made only 14 false responses.

The effects of lormetazepam and oxazepam on cognitive EPs

Figure 4 (left panel) illustrates the scalp distribution of EPs (for one of the naive subjects in a placebo run) for two types of cognitive stimuli, i.e., discrimination of amoeboid shapes and straight lines in terms of same or different. The RTs were recorded simultaneously. These discrimination tasks generated two prominent waves, i.e., the N200-P300 complex whose maximum was at the same location reported in other investigations (see Donchin, 1984). The trough-to-peak magnitude of this complex was taken as an EP measure of amplitude. P300 time to peak (latency) and RT comprised the other two parameters. The drug effects compared with placebo are shown at different times after ingestion of 45 mg oxazepam and 2 mg lormetazepam.

Figure 4 (top right) shows the plasma levels of 1 and 2 mg lormetazepam and of 45 mg oxazepam as a function of post-ingestion time, which serves here as a comparison of the drugs' neurophysiological effects. The results are the means for three subjects and show curves for conditions of stimulation/response (shapes—discrimination RT; lines—discrimination RT, and lines—simple

RT). The effects are shown as the percentage difference from the placebo condition. The following variables were normalized with respect to placebo: (a) dots P300 amplitude (b) squares—RT (two cognitive, one simple); and (c) stars—P300 latency (time to peak).

The first two factors show a greater percentage change than latency. Note that the percentage change is negative for P300, i.e., its size decreases, and positive for RT and latencies, i.e., an increase with drug action. The most significant effects of the drugs take place within four hours after lormetazepam ingestion, but the onset is much slower for oxazepam. The effects of lormetazepam are much more transient than those of oxazepam. In contrast, the effects of oxazepam are comparable with the plasma concentration.

Discussion

There are two main conclusions to be made here on the basis of the experiments with the task related potentials. First, the experimental conditions used are critical for the actual outcome. The investigator should aim to prevent fatigue and habituation which affect the size of EPs. When only unipolar recordings are available for analysis, great care has to be taken when selecting the stimulus parameters. The stimuli should be selective in that they should activate one rather than several neural systems. This is in reality not very easy to achieve, but certain measures such as the peripheral viewing applied in this study can selectively reduce the contribution of sensory components to the EP waveform and emphasize the cognitive elements. The various components can also be separated by computing Laplacean derivations but they must have different origins (see Kranda *et al.*, chapter 11, this volume).

False judgements seem to produce late components of undiminished amplitude, but the late waves seem somewhat broader (see Figure 3). Similar observations have been reported for false positive responses (i.e., response in the physical absence of the stimulus) provided the decisions were made with a high degree of confidence (Squires *et al.*, 1975). The significance of this similarity is, however, difficult to assess since a forced choice task was used in this study and the stimuli were always visible. Moreover, the subject had to discriminate between two shapes rather than having to indicate the simple presence or absence of a stimulus. Note that only correct detection of the location of grating stimuli seems to generate any wave (cf. Kranda *et al.*, chapter 11, in this volume). This inconsistency points to the difficulty of identifying the nature of the late components.

Secondly, the maximal reduction of the EP of about 30—40% occurs in the first three hours after lormetazepam ingestion, when the drug plasma concentration is still on the increase; the effect is much reduced when the plasma concentration levels off. This seemingly transient effect of the EPs is accompanied by a slightly more sustained increase in the RTs (Figure 4,

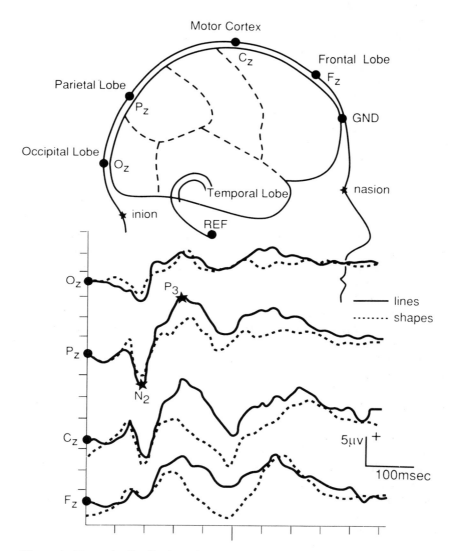

Figure 4. The scalp distribution of EPs produced by discrimination of amoeboid shapes (dotted) and lines (solid) for locations Oz, Pz, Cz, and Fz (the left panel). The right panel shows the time course of the concentration of oxazepam and lormetazepam in plasma and the time course of their effects on the amplitude and latency of P300 waves and the RTs expressed as a percentage difference with respect to placebo. The data have been averaged for four subjects.

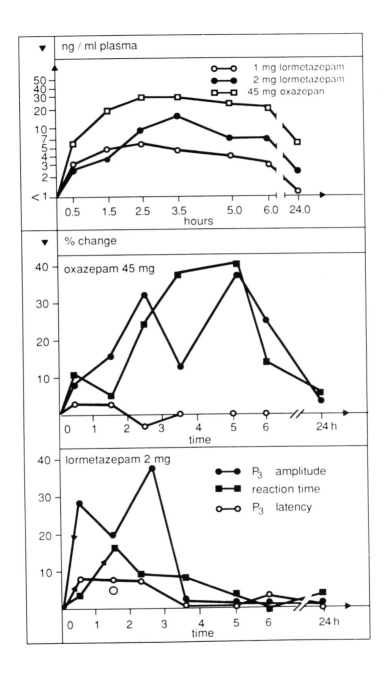

bottom). Note that a similar effect has been reported by Parry *et al.* (chapter 13, this volume). It appears that the dynamics of a drug effect do not always match the kinetics of the substance, and this indicates that knowledge of drug kinetics is insufficient for predicting the time course of the drug's actual neurophysiological action.

References

Ciesielski KT (1982) Lateralisation of visual cognitive potentials. *Biol. Psychol.* **14**, 259–70.

Ciesielski KT, Kulikowski JJ, Alvarez SL and Ott H (1983) The hangover effects of benzodiazepines on cognitive and visual functions. In: *Benzodiazepines, Sleep and Daytime Performance.* Oxford: Medicine Publishing Foundation.

Donchin E (1984) *Cognitive Psychology.* Hillsdale, New Jersey: Erlbaum

Hillyard SA and Kutas M (1983) Electrophysiology of cognitive processing. *Annu. Rev. Psychol.* **34**, 33–61.

Kulikowski JJ, McGlone F, Kranda K and Ott H (1984) Are the amplitudes of VEPs sensitive indices of hangover effects? In: *Sleep, Benzodiazepines and Performance* Hindmarch I, Ott H, and Roth T (eds.) pp. 154–164, Berlin: Springer Verlag.

Mackintosh N (1981) A new measure of intelligence. *Nature* **289**, 529–30.

Squires KC, Squires NK and Hillyard SA (1975) Decision-related cortical potentials during an auditory signal detection task with cued observation intervals. *Exp. Psychol: Hum. Percept. Perform.* **104**, 268–79.

Psychopharmacology and Reaction Time
Edited by I. Hindmarch, B. Aufdembrinke and H. Ott
© 1988 John Wiley & Sons Ltd

13

Visual Evoked Potentials and Reaction Times to Chromatic and Achromatic Stimulation: Psychopharmacological Applications

N. R. A. Parry[1], *J. J. Kulikowski*[1], *I. J. Murray*[1]*, *K. Kranda*[2], *and H. Ott*[2]

[1]*Visual Sciences Laboratory, University of Manchester Institute of Science and Technology, Manchester, UK*
[2]*Schering Research Laboratories, Berlin/Bergkamen, FRG*

General Introduction

The purpose of this chapter is to describe the development of a combined visual evoked potential and reaction time measure that can help us to compare the processing of chromatic and achromatic information in the human visual system. This technique has great potential when applied to the study of drug action.

We report that chromatic gratings generate visual evoked potentials (VEPs) that are distinctly different from VEPs to their achromatic counterparts (first part). We have also used chromatic gratings in a reaction-time (RT) task (second part). Finally, we introduce a procedure for testing the action of drugs on simultaneously recorded VEPs and RTs (third part). Before describing in detail the development of the test, some aspects of colour vision in the field of drug testing will briefly be reviewed, and the advantages of colour stimuli discussed.

*[*]I. J. Murray was supported by the Multiple Sclerosis Society of Great Britain and Northern Ireland.

Drugs and colour vision

As a result of recent progress in the study of colour vision and technical advances in the design of displays, the importance of colour as a stimulus parameter in the study of drug action has been recognized. Certain compounds have well-documented effects on colour vision, as illustrated by the following examples. Digoxin, a cardiac glycoside, is known to alter perception of colour (so-called 'yellow vision') when at toxic levels (e.g. Nimmo, 1979; Rietbrock and Alken, 1983). Lagerhof (1980) found colour deficiencies in 79% of rheumatic patients taking chloroquine and 57% of women taking oral contraceptives. Various colour vision defects are also associated with diabetes, alcohol poisoning and other conditions which induce retinal pathology (Birch *et al.*, 1980).

Investigation of drug action requires the separation of direct and indirect effects. When the effect of a compound on the central nervous system is studied, the choice of stimulus should ensure that the response is relatively immune to drug-induced changes in the peripheral nervous system. Two examples are the possible blurring of fine detail due to disturbance of accommodation and changes in retinal illumination due to fluctuations of pupil diameter.

Chromatic patterns have a clear advantage over achromatic patterns, since they can provide effective stimulation over a range of relatively low spatial frequencies (Granger and Heurtley, 1973; Mullen, 1985). Coarse patterns are not only less affected by optical distortion (Green and Campbell, 1965; Charman, 1983), but are generally easier to generate using conventional displays.

Visual Evoked Potentials to Colour Stimulation

The visual evoked potential (VEP) is an objective method of measuring brain activity related to a particular stimulus. It has been shown to be a powerful tool for investigating drug action (Zrenner, 1983), but the stimulus parameters have to be properly selected. For instance, it is difficult to separate the relative contribution to the VEP of different subsystems, such as those for processing pattern, colour or movement, when more than one subsystem is activated.

Early attempts to identify a VEP specific to colour used flash (rather than pattern) stimulation (Shipley *et al.*, 1965, 1966; Ciganek and Shipley, 1970; Kinney *et al.*, 1972; Yamanaka *et al.*, 1973), the responses to which were contaminated by a luminance increment. In some studies luminance changes were eliminated, leaving only pure hue changes (Regan, 1970, 1973a; Paulus *et al.*, 1984). However, the use of patterned stimuli seems preferable to that of nonstructured fields because the visual system, especially the visual cortex, contains cells that respond well to spatial and temporal changes (e.g. Hubel and Wiesel, 1959, 1968). Moreover, groupings of cells responding to changes in wavelength have been identified in the primate visual cortex (Michael, 1978; Livingstone and Hubel, 1984). In the cortex, a frequently encountered cell type is one that responds best to patches of light of long (red) and medium (green) wavelengths, presented in spatially adjacent areas (i.e. stimuli forming a chromatic border). This cell type does not respond to light of an intermediate wavelength that is neutral with respect to red and green (i.e. yellow—see Zrenner, 1983). We term such cells chromatic-opponent.

Responses of chromatic-opponent systems can be revealed psychophysically by testing threshold sensitivity with small stimuli (about $1°$ of visual angle) presented at a low temporal frequency (1 Hz) and superimposed on bright white backgrounds (Sperling and Harwerth, 1971; King-Smith, 1975). The spectral sensitivity curve obtained in these experiments can be considered to be an envelope of spectral characteristics of the chromatic-opponent mechanisms (see Sperling and Harwerth, 1971; King-Smith and Carden, 1976; Kranda and King-Smith, 1979). Zrenner (1983), using a similar paradigm, measured VEPs to coloured spots of different intensities and estimated their detection thresholds by extrapolating VEP amplitude to zero. These compared well with psychophysically measured chromatic opponent thresholds, in spite of the fact that flashed spots of high intensities probably also activated the achromatic (luminance) system.

Stimulation of the chromatic opponent system could be made more effective by using chromatic contours, with hues chosen to account for maximal wavelength discrimination (Butler and Riggs, 1978) or maximal chromatic contrast (Mullen, 1985).

Given these observations, an optimal stimulus for eliciting chromatic responses should comprise chromatic contours that are of equal luminance (isoluminant). Selected combinations of hues, e.g. red and green, may generate VEPs which reflect the activity of neural systems processing chromatic information (Hering, 1964). However, previous studies, generally using phase alternation (reversal) of chequer-board patterns, have showed little difference between VEPs to hue- and luminance-modulated stimuli (e.g. Regan, 1973b). The alternation of the pattern with a neutral field, with no change in space-averaged hue or luminance (onset presentation), might be expected to elicit much stronger changes in the total state of activity of the chromatic system than does phase alternation of the pattern. Regan and Spekreijse (1974), using chequer-board patterns, did not show any qualitative differences between VEPs to onset of chromatic and achromatic patterns. However, Carden *et al.* (1985), using sinusoidal gratings, generated using the method given below, described a clear difference between VEPs to onset of chromatic and achromatic patterns (a difference that was not revealed using reversal stimulation).

We have recently conducted a study using chequer-boards and gratings with both 15′ and 30′ elements. It is concluded that the chromatic-achromatic differences in VEP waveforms is revealed more effectively when gratings are used. (Kulikowski and Parry, 1987).

Method

Isoluminant red-green ('chromatic') sinusoidal gratings were produced on a colour monitor (Barco GD33). Video signals, derived from a BBC model B microcomputer, were modulated by two sinusoidal waves of opposite phase (see Figure 1). Isoluminance of the red-green pattern was determined, at all spatial frequencies, by heterochromatic flicker photometry; with adjacent stripes exchanging places at 25 Hz, the subject adjusted the relative luminance of the red and green components (without changing their contrast), until

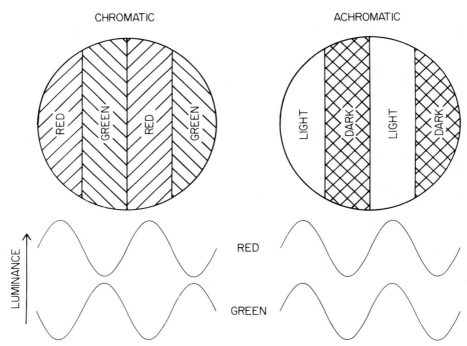

Figure 1. Diagrammatic representation of two cycles of a chromatic (red-green) grating and its achromatic (yellow−dark yellow) counterpart. As the luminance profiles below the gratings indicate, these sinusoidal patterns are generated by out-of-phase (chromatic) and in-phase (achromatic) superimposition of the component red and green sinusoidal patterns. In this system, these are combined electronically using an adding device. In onset/offset presentation mode, the pattern is replaced by a uniform yellow field, with no change in mean hue or space-averaged luminance; since these parameters are the same for both chromatic and achromatic patterns, their offsets are identical.

minimum flicker was observed. At this frequency, minimum flicker is observed only over a small range of red-green ratios. The red-green ratio at iso-luminance was found to be independent of spatial frequency. Conventional luminance-varying yellow ('achromatic') gratings were obtained by modulating the red and green video signals with two sinusoidal waves of equal phase. A plain yellow pattern offset was achieved by modulating the two video signals with unsynchronized high frequency (3 MHz) sinusoidal waves. Thus the red-green or the yellow-dark yellow gratings alternated with a uniform yellow field, without changing space-averaged hue or luminance. Manufacturers' quoted CIE chromaticity coordinates for the phosphors were $x = 0.61$, $y = 0.34$ (red) and $x = 0.28$, $y = 0.59$ (green).

Achromatic contrast (C) was defined according to Michelson as: $C = (L_{max} - L_{min})/(L_{max} + L_{min})$, where L_{max} and L_{min} are the luminances of the light and dark stripes respectively. Chromatic contrast cannot be unambiguously defined, due to the importance of two separate aspects. The first is physical: the contrast of a pattern with two spectral components is reduced as spectral overlap increases. The second is physiological, and here contrast depends on the mean physiological characteristics of the visual opponent mechanisms detecting chromatic differences. The simplest definition of chromatic contrast is that it is equivalent to the contrast of the two component gratings (if they are composed of monochromatic sources which correspond to the peak sensitivities of the opponent system, and have equal contrast— Mullen 1985). However, the phosphors of the display used here are not spectrally pure, since they have broad, overlapping, spectral emission curves. Since this inevitably reduces chromatic contrast, we introduced a correction factor of 0.56, or 0.25 log units. Thus a red-green grating generated by antiphase addition of red and green gratings of contrast 0.22 was assumed to have an equivalent chromatic contrast of 0.12. (This issue forms the basis of another study.)

VEPs were recorded with Ag/AgCl electrodes mounted on the scalp in standard positions based on the 10/20 system (Jasper, 1958). Recording electrodes were at the inion (In), mid-occipital (Oz) and mid-parietal (Pz) sites, and a point half-way between Oz and Pz (POz); these locations correspond to 0, 10, 30 and 20% of the inion–nasion distance. Linked ear electrodes served as reference, and a forehead electrode was grounded. The signals were amplified and averaged using a Medelec Sensor system (bandwidth 0.3–30 Hz), with an averaging epoch of 1000 msec and a stimulus duty cycle of 1040 msec. Each sweep was triggered by onset of the pattern. Data were stored on floppy disk, using an Apple IIe microcomputer. Hard copies were printed on a Hewlett-Packard HP7470A x-y plotter.

The display screen subtended $3°$ in diameter, and had a yellow surround. A cross in the centre of the display aided fixation. The subject was seated 172 cm from the screen. Viewing was binocular, since monocular viewing with an artificial pupil, employed in previous experiments, did not qualitatively alter the results. White acoustic noise was employed to mask relay sounds. The data presented here are for one subject (NRAP), age 30, with normal colour vision and normal visual acuity.

The effect of stimulus parameters on VEPs was examined with gratings having spatial frequencies of 1, 2, 4, 6 and 8 c/deg (cycles per degree of visual subtense), and the following onset and offset times: 260 msec on, 260 msec off; 260 msec on, 780 msec off; 60 msec on, 980 msec off.

The 4 c/deg, 760 msec on, 780 msec off data were repeated for 10 colour-normal subjects (8 males and 2 females, mean age 27.5 years), using central fixation of a 6° circular field. This larger field helps to overcome the poorer fixation of untrained subjects.

Results and comments

Figure 2 shows the effect of spatial frequency on VEPs elicited by colour-modulated (chromatic) and luminance-modulated (achromatic) gratings for

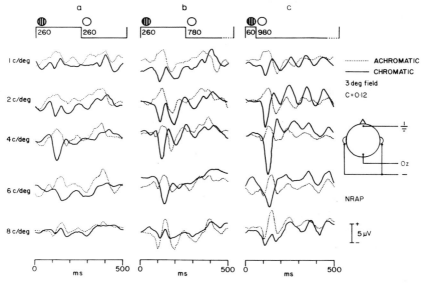

Figure 2. VEPs to onset of isoluminant red−green (chromatic) gratings (solid lines) and luminance-modulated yellow (achromatic) gratings (dotted lines), for a range of spatial frequencies (shown at left). Three degree (diameter) circular field, fixated centrally. $C = 0.12$. Mean luminance = 50 cd/m^2. Electrodes: Oz with linked-ears reference. 128 presentations. Averaging epoch 1000 msec (first 500 msec displayed here). Subject: NRAP. Stimulus timing: (a) onset 260 msec; offset 260 msec; (b) onset 260 msec; offset 780 msec; (c) onset 60 msec; offset 980 msec.

the three combinations of onset and offset times. Consider first the 260 msec on, 260 msec off condition (Figure 2a). The 'achromatic' onset wave is dominated by a prominent positive-going component with a time-to-peak of around 130 msec. On the other hand, the onset of the chromatic stimulus evokes, at moderate spatial frequencies (2–4 c/deg), a potential with a predominantly negative wave with approximately the same time-to-peak as the 'achromatic' positive wave. This fundamental difference between VEPs to achromatic and to chromatic patterns has been observed over a wide range of contrasts (0.08–0.2). The 'chromatic' VEP is attenuated at 6 c/deg and at 8 c/deg is hardly discernible from noise. This observation is consistent with psychophysical evidence from Mullen (1985), who reported that the red-green chromatic contrast sensitivity function declines rapidly for gratings finer than 6 c/deg, and also with our own measurements using gratings of broad-band spectral characteristics (Figure 3).

At the lowest spatial frequency (1 c/deg), the early negativity is less clear,

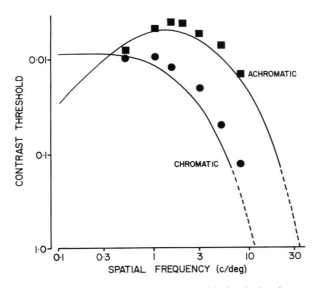

Figure 3. Detection contrast thresholds for isoluminant red–green (chromatic) gratings (circles) and luminance-modulated yellow (achromatic) gratings (squares), generated on a two-display set-up (to correct for chromatic aberrations), with phosphor characteristics approximating to those of the display used in the current study. Solid lines: chromatic (red–green) and achromatic (green) contrast sensitivity functions, from Mullen (1985), measured using two displays filtered to produce narrow-band spectral characteristics.

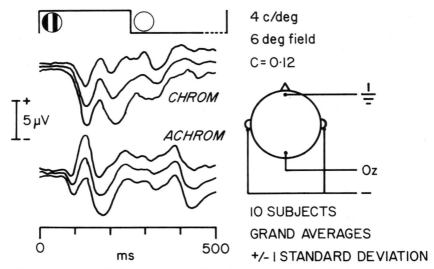

4 c/deg

6 deg field

C = O·l2

IO SUBJECTS

GRAND AVERAGES

+/- I STANDARD DEVIATION

Figure 4. Mean VEP waveforms elicited by onset of isoluminant red-green (chromatic) gratings (top) and luminance-modulated yellow (achromatic) gratings (bottom), plus and minus one standard deviation, for 10 subjects. Spatial frequency: 4 c/deg. 6° (diameter) circular field, fixated centrally. Mean luminance = 50 cd/m². Electrodes: Oz with linked-ears reference. 128 presentations. Averaging epoch 1000 msec (first 500 msec displayed here).

presumably because an achromatic component is also generated (note the presence of an offset wave, which is characteristic of an achromatic VEP).

Figure 2b shows the effect of increasing offset duration to 780 msec, whilst maintaining onset duration at 260 msec. The difference between 'chromatic' and 'achromatic' waveforms is still most pronounced at 4 c/deg, but is much clearer than before at 1 c/deg, probably because the long offset allows greater recovery from adaptation.

Figure 2c demonstrates that the onset duration of 60 msec merely serves to enhance the negative component of the 'chromatic' VEP, indicating that this kind of presentation is suitable for VEP studies. (Note that short durations are preferred in reaction time studies.)

Figure 4 gives an indication of the degree of repeatability of the fundamental effect we describe here. Ten subjects' VEPs were recorded to 4 c/deg chromatic and achromatic gratings, using an onset time of 260 msec and an offset time of 780 msec. Waveforms were normalized with respect to the mean DC level of their first 66 msec, and average VEPs computed. These are displayed in Figure 4, plus and minus one standard deviation.

The pronounced difference between the two waveforms allows us to study chromatic and achromatic responses at low to moderate spatial frequencies.

The relatively simple negative-going waveform may reflect the specificity of the stimulus, representing the activity of neurons which share similar response properties, and which may be located in a specific region of the brain. Russell *et al.* (1986) recorded similar VEP waveforms to very fine achromatic gratings (up to 30 c/deg), which are known to be detected predominantly by the part of the striate cortex representing central (foveal) vision; in man, this representation is near the tip of the occiput (Holmes, 1918). Macaque field potential studies have demonstrated that, when a functionally homogeneous population of cells is activated, the response takes a simple, negative-going form (Russell *et al.*, 1986; Kulikowski and Vidyasagar, 1986).

Reaction Times to Coloured Stimuli

Investigations of reaction times (RTs) to chromatic stimulation have rarely been specifically designed with the aim of separating the response of chromatic and achromatic systems but were more concerned with the effect of wavelength, without controlling luminance. The results of such experiments were inconsistent (see for instance Pollack, 1968; Lit *et al.*, 1971; Mollon and Krauskopf, 1973; Koslow, 1984). Subsequent investigations were more analytical in trying to test selectively the response of chromatic and achromatic detection systems (Regan and Tyler, 1971; Nissen and Pokorny, 1977). However, the problems concerning result comparability remained, largely because of the investigators' inability to define the relative sensitivities of the detection systems (both chromatic and achromatic) for given experimental conditions. One approach which has allowed the separation of chromatic and achromatic systems is to examine the temporal distribution of near-threshold RTs by constructing histograms (c.f. Schwartz and Loop, 1982; Kranda, 1983). Yet the different spatial parameters of the stimuli used by Schwartz and Loop (1982) and by Kranda (1983) have produced apparently contradictory results regarding the temporal characteristics of the achromatic detection system. This controversy can, however, be reconciled if one considers the possibility that the achromatic detection system can behave in a sustained as well as in a transient manner (c.f. Tolhurst, 1975; Kranda, 1985).

Using suprathreshold gratings of moderate spatial frequency, Harwerth and Levi (1978) showed that the plot of RT as a function of contrast is biphasic, in that it consists of two distinct branches. This indicates that mechanisms with different temporal characteristics dominate the response at high and low contrasts. It is important to characterize the contrast relationship of RTs to red-green gratings, if these are to be used in clinical trials. We describe below an experiment designed to compare RT-versus-contrast function for achromatic and chromatic gratings.

Methods

A modification to the stimulator allowed the measurement of RTs. A hardware timer, with a resolution of 1 msec, was connected to the microcomputer's 1 MHz bus. The timer was started by stimulus onset and stopped by the subject, who was instructed to respond to the appearance of the grating by pressing a microswitch, as rapidly as possible, with his right index finger. The grating, presented for 60 msec, was followed by a uniform field (offset) whose duration varied in the following manner. Once the subject had responded (or after a default period of 2000 msec, if no response was made), an additional offset period followed. The length of this was varied randomly, such that there was an equal probability of the subsequent stimulus appearing at the end of any 20 msec period between 1000 msec and 3000 msec after the response (or after the default period). All raw RTs were stored on disk for later analysis, although those of less than 150 msec or greater than 1000 msec were not analysed. RTs were determined for a range of contrasts. Expressed in log units, achromatic contrasts (see also previous section) were $-0.6, -1.7, -0.8, -0.9, -1.0, -1.1, -1.2, -1.3, -1.4, -1.5, -1.6$ and -1.7; chromatic contrasts were $-0.55, -0.65, -0.85, -0.9, -0.95$ and -1.05. Different contrasts were presented in blocks of 25 trials, ascending and descending through the range twice. Hence 100 RTs were collected at each contrast level. A block of 25 RTs took approximately 90 sec to collect.

The subject (MHAR) was a colour vision-normal male, age 27, with normal visual acuity when corrected. He was well practised, having had at least 30 hours experience of the RT procedure. He was, however, unaware of the exact purpose of this experiment.

Results and comments

Figure 5 shows mean RT plotted as a function of contrast for achromatic (squares) and chromatic (circles) 2 c/deg gratings. The curve for RTs to achromatic gratings has two branches, as though different mechanisms (or combinations of mechanisms) were activated and determined the response at high and at low contrasts·(see also Harwerth and Levi, 1978, for similar results). From neurophysiological findings, we know that achromatic gratings whose contrast is less than about 0.1 activate only the phasic system (Kaplan and Shapley, 1982; Hicks *et al.*, 1983). The RT/contrast function for chromatic gratings does not appear to show the branching seen in its achromatic counterpart. The RTs to chromatic gratings are clearly longer than those for achromatic stimulation, which is consistent with the slower response of the chromatic system as known from the neurophysiology of tonic cells (e.g. Gouras, 1969; Dreher *et al.*, 1976; Marrocco, 1976). The different slopes of

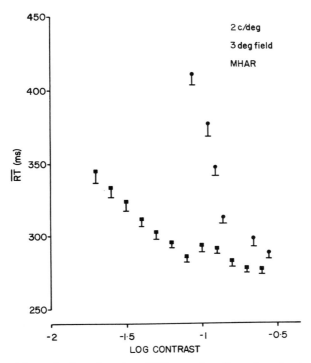

Figure 5. Reaction time (RT) as a function of contrast for isoluminant red–green (chromatic) gratings (circles) and luminance-modulated yellow (achromatic) gratings (squares). Means and SE of 128 trials. Spatial frequency: 2 c/deg. 3° (diameter) circular field, fixated centrally. Mean luminance = 50 cd/m². Onset duration: 60 msec. Time between response and next stimulus: 1000–3000 msec (random). Subject: MHAR.

the two functions presumably reflect the higher contrast threshold for red-green gratings of this spatial frequency (c.f. Figure 3).

Parallel VEP and Reaction Time Studies—A Two-dimensional Approach to Drug Testing

In the first two sections, we have singled out suitable electrophysiological and behavioural techniques for comparing the processing of achromatic and chromatic signals. Here we combine the two techniques in one experiment by recording VEPs during a reaction time task. This approach enables us effectively to double the information available without increasing experimental time. This economy of time is particularly important if we wish to follow the kinetics of drug action.

In order successfully to combine VEPs and RTs in a single paradigm, it is firstly necessary to ensure that interaction between the tasks is minimized. This problem is considered first. Secondly, a range of stimulus parameters that suit both VEPs and RTs must be chosen, and the extent to which they covary across this range examined.

Effect of passive and active conditions on the VEP waveform

One of the recurring themes of this chapter has been the need to find a stimulus which specifically activates a given neural centre. It is important to ascertain that the VEP components related purely to sensory mechanisms are not distorted by the subject's involvement in a parallel RT task, or by overlapping the response-related components of the VEP. If these two factors can be dissociated, it may be possible to obtain and analyse additional task-related VEPs.

Methods

There were two experimental conditions: passive (VEPs only) and active (simultaneous VEPs and RTs). In the passive condition, the subject fixated the screen, as in the experiment described in the first section, but did not respond. In the active condition, the subject responded, as he did in the experiment described in the second section.

The stimulus configuration and timing were the same as before (see second section) except that, in the passive condition, the default period was reduced from 2000 msec to 300 msec. Thus the inter-stimulus interval was between 1300 msec and 3300 msec. VEPs were recorded from Pz, POz, Oz and Inion, with linked-ears reference. The averaging epoch was 1000 msec. The subject was MHAR (see second section).

Results and comments

Figure 6 shows chromatic VEPs recorded at four midline electrodes (Pz, POz, Oz and Inion), under conditions of either passive viewing (left) or active response to the gratings (right). In the passive condition, the VEP is a simple negative-going wave (c.f. Figure 2). Its amplitude is maximal at Oz, which is positioned just above the tip of the visual cortex. In the active condition, an additional slow positive-going wave, which peaks at around 350 msec and is maximal at Pz, is evident. This 'pseudo-cognitive' wave (often called P300) signals the subject's active involvement in the task. These two components can be separated since they have different latencies and their sources have different locations. This is not generally the case with VEPs to coarse achromatic gratings, since they tend to interact with P300 (see McGlone *et al.*, chapter 12,

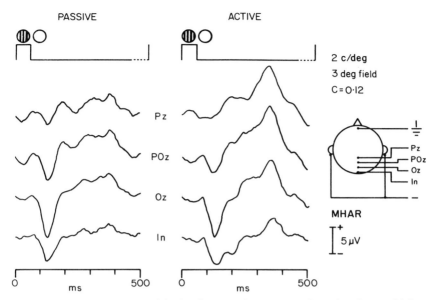

Figure 6. VEPs to onset of isoluminant red–green gratings for four mid-line electrodes (Inion, Oz, POz and Pz) with linked-ears reference. Spatial frequency: 2 c/deg. $C = 0.12$. 3° (diameter) circular field, fixated centrally. Mean luminance = 50 cd/m². 128 presentations. Averaging epoch: 1000 msec (first 500 msec displayed here). Subject: MHAR.

Left column (passive): no secondary task. Stimulus timing: onset 60 msec; offset 1300–3300 msec (random).

Right column (active): recorded whilst subject performed simultaneous RT task (responding to grating onset). Stimulus timing: onset 60 msec; Time between response and next stimulus: 1000–3000 msec (random). Note the difference in the scalp distribution of the early negativity (N1) and the late positivity (P300).

this volume). Moreover, because the subject has to respond to the appearance of each grating the investigator has some index of the subject's attention—an important consideration in most drug studies.

Effect of contrast on simultaneous VEPs and RTs

There have been many attempts to correlate VEP latencies (or, more precisely, times to peak for various VEP components) with reaction times (RTs) for a range of stimulus parameters, e.g. spatial frequency and contrast. The main line of argument was that VEP timing is related mainly to grating detectability and varies little with spatial frequency of the gratings when appropriate corrections for equal suprathreshold contrast are made (see Kulikowski, 1977). Musselwhite and Jeffreys (1985) have recently re-examined this prob-lem, and compared the measurements of VEPs and RTs. They pointed out that apparently large increases in latency of VEP with spatial frequency often result from the inability to identify individual VEP components. In their experiments, the first component, C1, had latencies independent of spatial frequency, whereas RT tended to increase with spatial frequency (see also Kranda *et al.*, chapter 11, this volume). Here we reaffirm that the VEP latencies and RTs are different functions of contrast when obtained in the same experimental session.

Methods

The stimulus configuration and timing were the same as in the experiment described in the second section. Eight contrast levels were used (expressed in log units, these were: -0.65, -0.7, -0.75, -0.8, -0.85, -0.95, -1.05 and -1.15). Different contrasts were presented in blocks of 32 trials, ascending and descending through the range twice. The subject was given a one minute break between each block. The whole experiment comprised 128 individual reaction times and 128 VEP sweeps for each contrast. Eight VEP files were set up on the Apple microcomputer, one for each contrast, and could be recalled to the averager so that further sweeps could be added. Electrode montage was the same as in experiments described in the first section. The duration of the experimental session was approximately 90 min. The subject was MHAR (see second section) who, again, was not informed as to the purpose of the experiment.

Results and comments

Figure 7 summarizes data from simultaneously recorded VEPs and RTs to gratings of different chromatic contrasts. The VEP waveforms are similar to those shown in Figure 6 (right). Amplitudes and latencies (times-to-peak) of the negative 'chromatic' wave (N1) and the 'cognitive' wave (referred to as P300) were measured using the VEPs derived from locations Oz and Pz respectively. These results are plotted along with mean RT. The parameters of the regression lines for these data are given in Table 1.

It appears that the latencies to 'chromatic' (N1) and 'cognitive' (P300) EP components vary much less with contrast than mean RT (note their different slopes). RTs increase with decreasing contrast (c.f. Figure 5 and note that the scales for Figure 5 and 7 are different). It seems unlikely that the latency increase of the two EP components can account for the increase of mean RTs. Note also that the latencies of P300 and N1 are shifted by an almost constant amount (in that they have similar slopes with means separated by 230 msec), as though the cognitive wave was delayed only by the delayed sensory event. It is interesting that, unlike the early VEP components, the amplitude of the 'cognitive' P300 component is virtually independent of contrast: the slope of the regression of P300 amplitude on contrast does not differ significantly from zero ($t = -0.595$, d.f. $= 6$), whereas that for N1 amplitude on contrast is

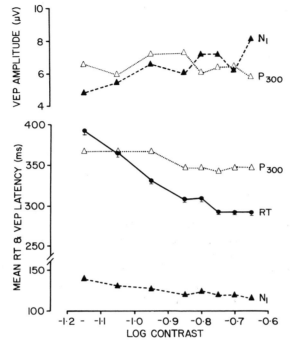

Figure 7. Mean RT (+SE), latency (time-to-peak) of two VEP components (P300 = late positive wave — see Figure 6, right column; N1 = 'chromatic' early negativity), as a function of contrast. Stimulus was onset of an isoluminant red-green grating, spatial frequency 2 c/deg. Three degree (diameter) circular field, fixated centrally. Mean luminance = 50 cd/m². Electrodes: Oz with linked-ears reference. 128 presentations. VEPs and RTs recorded simultaneously. Stimulus timing: onset 60 msec; time between response and next stimulus: 1000–3000 msec (random). Subject: MHAR. The lines are only provided to guide the eye. Note the break in the ordinate.

Table 1. Parameters of the regression lines fitted to the data in Figure 7

Relationship correlation between log contrast and	Central point			Regression		
	x mean	*y* mean	*y* SD	Slope	SD	*r*
N1 AMP (μV)	− 0.86	6.43	1.07	5.08	1.39	0.83
P300 AMP (μV)	− 0.86	6.45	0.55	− 0.74	1.24	− 0.24
RT (msec)	− 0.86	323.38	37.40	− 207.31	21.73	− 0.97
N1 LAT (msec)	− 0.86	125.00	7.93	− 43.51	5.25	− 0.96
P300 LAT (msec)	− 0.86	355.00	10.85	− 54.74	11.96	− 0.88

significantly greater than zero ($P < 0.01$, $t = 3.659$, d.f. = 6). Thus all these variables appear to be different functions of contrast, thereby providing possibly complementary information.

Effect of lormetazepam on chromatic and achromatic VEPs and RTs

Earlier studies carried out in this laboratory (Ciesielski *et al.*, 1983; Kulikowski *et al.*, 1984) have shown that effects of benzodiazepines are manifested by increased RTs and reduced amplitudes of both cognitive and achromatic (grating onset) VEPs. The latencies in these experiments were unaffected. VEPs to passively viewed gratings, presented at a rate of 2 Hz, showed larger amplitude reduction for finer (8 c/deg) than coarser (2 c/deg) gratings. This effect on VEP amplitude could reflect poor fixation or accommodation which may degrade the retinal image. One reason for this may have been the sleepiness of the subject. This latter problem can be alleviated by adding an RT task, even though the testing time would be prolonged due to the lower presentation rate (below 1 Hz). Moreover, the use of relatively coarse chromatic stimuli offers an additional advantage over fine gratings since the VEPs elicited by chromatic gratings contain a simple negative wave that considerably differs from the positive P300.

Methods

In this experiment, simultaneous VEPs and RTs were recorded for chromatic and achromatic 2 c/deg gratings. A larger screen (6° diameter) and relatively high contrast ($C = 0.18$ or -0.75 log units) were chosen, so that VEP amplitudes are large, and the vulnerability of RT to fluctuations in contrast is minimized (see Figures 5 and 7). The disadvantages of this choice are, however, (a) that the cognitive wave may be small compared with the early VEP components, and (b) reduced selectivity of stimulation of chromatic and achromatic mechanisms (since at high contrasts involvement of several mechanisms cannot be excluded). The effects of contrast and stimulus configuration are the subjects of further investigation. Stimulus timing was as described in the second section. RTs and VEPs were averaged over 128 presentations. Data collection took approximately 12 minutes for one chromatic and one achromatic run, and this was repeated approximately every 30 minutes for 4.5 hours. This procedure was repeated on two consecutive days. On the first day, the subject ingested a placebo after the second run. On the second, he ingested 2 mg lormetazepam (Noctamid). Precise timing of the experiments can be seen in Figure 8. The subject was MHAR (see second section). The procedure was single-blind, since the subject was informed that he would receive two doses of the drug, but not on which day he would receive the higher dose, nor that one of the doses was a placebo. The data described have been replicated using one of the authors (NRAP) as subject.

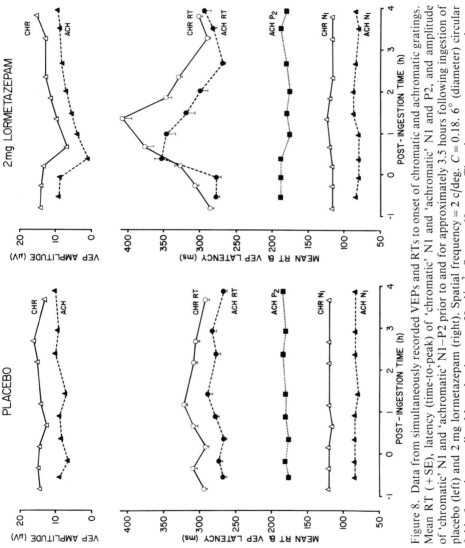

Figure 8. Data from simultaneously recorded VEPs and RTs to onset of chromatic and achromatic gratings. Mean RT (+SE), latency (time-to-peak) of 'chromatic' N1 and 'achromatic' N1 and P2, and amplitude of 'chromatic' N1 and 'achromatic' N1–P2 prior to and for approximately 3.5 hours following ingestion of placebo (left) and 2 mg lormetazepam (right). Spatial frequency = 2 c/deg. $C = 0.18$. $6°$ (diameter) circular field, fixated centrally. Mean luminance = 50 cd/m^2. Onset = 60 msec; Time between response and next stimulus = 1000–3000 msec (random), 128 presentations per data point. Subject: MHAR.

Results and comments

Figure 8 shows VEP amplitude and latency and mean RT for chromatic and achromatic gratings, measured over a period of 4.5 hours for placebo (left) and drug (right) conditions. The amplitudes of both VEPs are reduced following ingestion of the lormetazepam, this reduction being greatest between 20 and 40 minutes after administration of the drug. The placebo condition shows only small, apparently random, variations during the same period. RTs are increased markedly following ingestion of the drug, whilst only relatively minor fluctuations are seen during the placebo condition. Latencies to the negative component (N1) of the 'chromatic' VEP and to two components (the early negativity, N1 and the late positivity, P2) of the 'achromatic' VEP do not seem to vary systematically under placebo or lormetazepam.

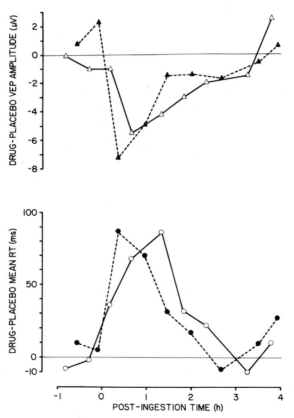

Figure 9. VEP amplitudes and mean RT from Figure 8, plotted in terms of drug data minus placebo data, as a function of post-ingestion time.

In order to express more clearly the effect on VEP amplitude and RT following ingestion of the drug, Figure 9 shows the result of subtracting placebo data from drug data, this difference being plotted as a function of post-ingestion time. It can be seen that there may be a somewhat earlier effect of lormetazepam on achromatic VEPs and RTs than on their chromatic equivalents. Despite this, the effects are generally similar, and are consistent with the non-specificity of action of this benzodiazepine, in that it reduces the responses of systems processing both chromatic and achromatic visual information. This reflects the distribution of GABA-ergic receptors in the visual cortex: these receptors are found both inside patches labelled by cytochrome oxidase, which are the sites of neurons processing chromatic information, as well as outside these patches, where neurons process achromatic contrast (Livingstone and Hubel, 1984).

Concluding Remarks

The method presented in this study allows the simultaneous recording of reaction times and averaged occipital potentials evoked by onset of patterns which are isoluminant chromatic (red-green) or luminance-modulated (yellow). Mean reaction time and evoked potential amplitude are convenient measures of response; they are different functions of fundamental stimulus parameters such as contrast, and they reflect the contribution of different neuronal mechanisms. Using this technique, the degree of selectivity of various factors on chromatic and achromatic mechanisms can be studied. Our preliminary results do not indicate strong selectivity of lormetazepam, except possibly for some degree of temporal shift.

Acknowledgements

The authors would like to express their gratitude to Dave Carden and John Simpson for their invaluable assistance, and to Martyn Russell for the many hours he spent as a subject.

References

Birch J, Hamilton AM and Gould ES (1980) Colour vision in relation to the clinical features and extent of field loss in diabetic retinopathy. In: Verriest G (ed). *Colour Vision Deficiencies V*. pp. 83–88, Bristol: Adam Hilger.

Butler TW and Riggs LA (1978) Color differences scaled by chromatic modulation sensitivity functions. *Vision Res.* **18**, 1407–16.

Carden D, Kulikowski JJ, Murray IJ and Parry NRA (1985) Human occipital potentials evoked by the onset of equiluminant chromatic gratings. *J. Physiol. (Lond.)* **369**, 44.

Ciesielski KT, Kulikowski JJ, Kranda K, Alvarez SL and Ott H (1983) The hangover effects of benzodiazepines on cognitive and visual functions. In: *Benzodiazepines, Sleep and Daytime Performance*. Oxford: The Medicine Publishing Foundation.

Charman WN (1983) The retinal image in the human eye. In: Osborne N and Chader G (eds). *Progress in Retinal Research Vol 2*. pp. 1–50, Oxford: Pergamon.

Ciganek L and Shipley T (1970) Color evoked brain responses in man. *Vision Res.* **10**, 917–9.

Dreher B, Fukada Y and Rodiek RW (1976) Identification, classification and anatomical segregation of cells with X-like and Y-like properties in the lateral geniculate nucleus of old-world primates. *J. Physiol. (Lond.)* **258**, 433–52.

Gouras P (1969) Antidromic responses of orthodromically identified ganglion cells in monkey retina. *J. Physiol. (Lond.)* **204**, 407–19.

Granger EM and Heurtley JC (1973) Visual chromaticity modulation transfer function. *J. Opt. Soc. Am.* **63**, 73–4.

Green DG and Campbell FW (1965) Effect of focus on the visual response to a sinusoidally modulated spatial stimulus. *J. Opt. Soc. Am.* **55**, 1154–7.

Harwerth RS and Levi DM (1978) Reaction time as a measure of suprathreshold grating detection. *Vision Res.* **18**, 1579–86.

Hering E (1964) Outlines of a theory of the light sense. (Translated by Hurvich LM and Jameson D). Cambridge, Mass: Harvard University Press.

Hicks TP, Lee BB and Vidyasagar TR (1983) The responses of cells in macaque lateral geniculate nucleus to sinusoidal gratings. *J. Physiol. (Lond.)* **337**, 183–200.

Holmes G (1918) Disturbances of vision by cerebral lesions. *Br. J. Ophthalmol.* **2**, 353–84.

Hubel DH and Wiesel TN (1959) Receptive fields of single neurones in the cat striate cortex. *J. Physiol. (Lond.)* **148**, 574–91.

Hubel DH and Wiesel TN (1968) Receptive fields and functional architecture of monkey striate cortex. *J. Physiol. (Lond.)* **195**, 215–43.

Jasper HH (1958) Report of a committee on methods of examination in electro-encephalography. *Electroencephalogr. Clin. Neurophysiol.* **10**, 370–5.

Kaplan E and Shapley RM (1982) X and Y cells in the lateral geniculate nucleus of macaque monkeys. *J. Physiol. (Lond.)* **330**, 125–43.

King-Smith PE (1975) Visual detection analysed in terms of luminance and chromatic signals. *Nature* **255**, 69–70.

King-Smith PE and Carden D (1976) Luminance and opponent-color contributions to visual detection and adaptation and to temporal and spatial integration. *J. Opt. Soc. Am.* **66**, 709–17.

Kinney JAS, McKay CL, Mensch AJ and Luria SM (1972) Techniques for analysing differences in VERs: coloured and patterned stimuli. *Vision Res.* **12**, 1733–47.

Koslow RE (1984) Reaction times as related to ball color. *Percept. Motor Skills* **57**, 871–4.

Kranda K (1983) Analysis of reaction times to coloured stimuli. *Ophthal. Physiol. Optics* **3**, 223–31.

Kranda K (1985) On reaction time histograms: Reply to Schwartz. *Ophthalmic Physiol. Opt.* **5**, 225–6.

Kranda K and King-Smith PE (1979) Detection of coloured stimuli by independent linear systems. *Vision Res.* **19**, 733–45.

Kulikowski JJ (1977) Visual evoked potentials as a measure of visibility. In: Desmedt JE (ed) *Visual Evoked Potentials in Man: New Developments*. pp. 168–183, Oxford: Clarendon Press.

Kulikowski JJ, McGlone FF, Kranda K and Ott H (1984) Are the amplitudes of visual evoked potentials sensitive indices of hangover effects after repeated doses of benzodiazepines? In: Hindmarch I, Ott H and Roth T (eds) *Sleep, Benzodiazepines and Performance*. Berlin: Springer-Verlag.

Kulikowski JJ and Parry NRA (1987) Human occipital potentials evoked by achromatic or chromatic checkerboards and gratings. *J. Physiol. (Lond.)* **388**, 45.

Kulikowski JJ and Vidyasagar TR (1986) Space and spatial frequency: Analysis and representation in the macaque striate cortex. *Exp. Brain Res.* **64**, 5–19.

Lagerhof O (1980) Drug-induced colour vision deficiencies. In: Verriest G (ed). Colour Vision Deficiencies V. pp. 317–319, Bristol: Adam Hilger.

Lit A, Young RH and Shaffer M (1971) Simple time reaction as a function of luminance for various wavelengths. *Perception and Psychophysics* **10**, 397–9.

Livingstone MS and Hubel DH (1984) Anatomy and physiology of a color system in the primate visual cortex. *J. Neurosci.* **4**, 309–56.

Marrocco RT (1976) Sustained and transient cells in monkey lateral geniculate nucleus: Conduction velocities and response properties. *J. Neurophysiol.* **39**, 340–53.

Michael CR (1978) Colour vision mechanisms in monkey striate cortex: Dual opponent cells with concentric receptive fields. *J. Neurophysiol.* **41**, 572–88.

Mollon JD and Krauskopf J (1973) Reaction time as a measure of the temporal response properties of individual colour mechanisms. *Vision Res.* **13**, 27–40.

Mullen KT (1985) The contrast sensitivity of human colour vision to red-green and blue-yellow chromatic gratings. *J. Physiol. (Lond.)* **359**, 381–400.

Musselwhite MJ and Jeffreys DA (1985) The influence of spatial frequency on the reaction times and evoked potentials recorded to grating pattern stimuli. *Vision Res.* **25**, 1545–55.

Nimmo J (1979) Drugs acting on the cardiovascular system. In: Girdwood RH (ed). *Clin. Pharmacol.* 24e. London: Baillière Tindall.

Nissen MJ and Pokorny J (1977) Wavelength effects on simple reaction time. *Perception and Psychophysics* **22**, 457–62.

Paulus WM, Homberg V, Cunningham K, Halliday AM and Rohde N (1984) Colour and brightness components of foveal visual evoked potentials in man. *Electroencephalogr. Clin. Neurophysiol.* **58**, 107–19.

Pollack JD (1968) Reaction time to different wavelengths at various luminances. *Perception and Psychophysics* **3**, 17–24.

Regan D (1970) Evoked potential and psychophysical correlates of changes in stimulus colour and intensity. *Vision Res.* **10**, 163–78.

Regan D (1973a) An evoked potential correlate of colour: Evoked potential findings and single-cell speculations. *Vision Res.* **13**, 1933–41.

Regan D (1973b) Evoked potentials specific to spatial patterns of luminance and colour. *Vision Res.* **13**, 2381–402.

Regan D and Spekreijse J (1974) Evoked potential indications of colour blindness. *Vision Res.* **14**, 89–95.

Regan D and Tyler CW (1971) Some dynamic features of colour vision. *Vision Res.* **11**, 1307–24.

Rietbrock N and Alken RG (1983) Color vision deficiencies: A common sign of intoxication in chronically digoxin-treated patients. In: Verriest G (ed). *Colour Vision Deficiencies V*. pp. 59–65, Bristol: Adam Hilger.

Russell MHA, Kulikowski JJ, Parry NRA, Murray IJ and Stafford CA (1986) Negative occipital potential evoked by onset of fine gratings. *Electroencephalogr. Clin. Neurophysiol.* **63**, 80.

Schwartz SH and Loop MS (1982) Evidence for transient luminance and quasi-sustained color mechanisms. *Vision Res.* **22**, 445–7.

Shipley T, Jones RW and Fry A (1965) Evoked visual potentials and human color vision. *Science* **150**, 1162–4.

Shipley T, Jones RW and Fry A (1966) Intensity and the evoked occipitogram in man. *Vision Res.* **6**, 657–67.

Sperling HG and Harwerth RS (1971) Red-green cone interaction in the incremental threshold spectral sensitivity of primates. *Science* **172**, 180–4.

Tolhurst DJ (1975) Reaction times in the detection of gratings by human observers: A probabilistic mechanism. *Vision Res.* **15**, 1143–9.

Yamanaka T, Sobagaki H and Nayatani Y (1973) Opponent-colors response in the visually evoked potential in man. *Vision Res.* **13**, 1319–33.

Zrenner E (1983) *Neurophysiological Aspects of Color Vision in Primates.* Berlin: Springer-Verlag.

Psychopharmacology and Reaction Time
Edited by I. Hindmarch, B. Aufdembrinke and H. Ott
© 1988 John Wiley & Sons Ltd

14

Explaining the Common Effect of Sedative Drugs on Driving using Performance Models: Concepts and a Research Plan

James F. O'Hanlon

Institute for Drugs, Safety and Behaviour, State University of Limburg, Maastricht, The Netherlands

Abstract

Repeated experiments have demonstrated a common effect of many types of sedative drugs (anxiolytics, antidepressants, antihistamines, hypnotics, and ethanol) on actual driving performance in a standard test. Specifically, the drugs caused the drivers to allow a rise in their vehicle's lateral position variability during high-speed uninterrupted travel. This appears to be a robust and reliable effect, but until now it has not been interpreted to reveal the underlying source of the impairment.

Strictly pharmacological interpretations seem largely pointless, because the drugs' known mechanisms of action often differ greatly within the same therapeutic categories, and nearly always between different categories. An alternative approach is to examine the common effect in terms of models of human road-tracking performance. Several such models are examined in turn, all of which offer plausible explanations for the observed effect of sedative drugs. The respective explanations depend, however, upon different assumptions regarding the impaired psychological processes and cannot all be correct.

A research programme is therefore proposed for testing their validity with respect to a number of phenomena that are associated with, but not the same as, the observed effect. A successful conclusion of such a programme might not only reveal the final common path mediating the influence of all sedative drugs on driving performance, but also indicate which model is likely to be valid in a general sense.

Introduction

We have repeatedly observed a common effect of many sedative drugs (tranquilizers, antidepressants, hypnotics, and ethanol (O'Hanlon, 1986)) on actual driving performance during high-speed uninterrupted vehicle operation. The drugs adversely affect the drivers' ability to control their vehicle's lateral position while they attempt to steer a straight course between traffic lane boundaries. Side-to-side motion increases until it assumes proportions commonly described as 'weaving'. In extreme cases, this has forced discontinuation of the test after less than one hour. In all of our studies, lateral position relative to painted lane markers was recorded continuously and automatically with a special electro-optical device. Afterwards, the recordings were analysed to yield a single measure of control precision: the standard deviation (SD) of lateral position over segments of the total distance travelled (usually 100 km).

The measure is easily understood and is relevant to safety, since an increasing SD of lateral position relates in an entirely predictable manner to the crossing of lane boundaries once the data are adjusted for mean position, skew, and kurtosis. This measure reveals nothing, however, of the psychophysiological processes or their functional impairment that must underlie the observed performance changes. It is thus a measure of limited theoretical importance.

For a while we were content to establish merely the reliability and generality of this phenomenon and to use the measure for comparing different drugs in relation to their known pharmacokinetics and dynamics. Now may be the time to search for the process whose impairment by many different types of sedative drugs could be responsible for their common behavioural effect. Purely pharmacological considerations are of little help, since the known mechanisms of action differ widely between the various drugs studied to date. Either pharmacological mechanisms of action operate at a lower level than the one responsible, as the final common path, for mediating the behavioural effect, or there is some as yet unknown mechanism of action on a higher level that is shared by all sedative drugs. Whatever the case may be, it seems more fruitful to approach the question through the application of performance models which have been developed to explain the manual vehicle control under circumstances similar to those of the test. Inferences and the selective exclusion of unlikely alternatives could isolate a number of hypothetical psychological processes whose impairment could be responsible for the behavioural effect.

Every modern model represents the human operator as a servocontrol system, continuously or intermittently active. Multiple perceptual error signals are the system's input, and motor responses affecting steering-wheel movement are the output. This response translates through the dynamics of the vehicle-road system into a new pattern of error signals to complete the feedback loop. The functional relationship between the operator's input and output is specified by the particular model's variables so as to determine amplitude, frequency, and other temporal characteristics of road tracking performance.

Every variable represents, either explicitly or implicitly, a particular brain process. Examples are neuromuscular delay lag and system gain, conceived as a phasic activation process and information sampling rate. Exercising a model by systematically varying the value of one variable while holding the others constant produces a characteristic effect on the system's output. When the effects are similar to those produced by a sedative drug, one can infer that the associated process is among those capable of being influenced by the drug.

A rigorous and exhaustive study of each performance model's utility for describing the observed sedative effects on SD lateral position is beyond the scope of this chapter. Several of the most popular, or most recent, models will be examined in turn to determine whether this approach has any promise for explaining the observed phenomena.

The Crossover Model

McRuer and coworkers introduced and subsequently refined the crossover model of tracking performance (McRuer and Weir, 1969; McRuer *et al.* 1975; Weir and McRuer, 1968; 1973). Mathematically rigorous and conceptually simple, this model has numerous successful applications and has served as the point of departure for nearly all subsequent models of tracking performance.

In this model, the driver responds to a composite heading angle and lateral position error (Ψ_a) by moving a steering wheel (δ_w), which effects a compensatory change in the vehicle's turning rate. The driver thus behaves as a first-order system controller by integrating the error signal over time to effect a change in the vehicle's angular velocity.

Only two variables determine the relationship between the perceptual input and the motor output in the simplest case of straight road and compensatory tracking. The first is gain, K, which determines the amplitude of output relative to input. The second is pure time delay or driver transmission lag, τ, which is analogous to reaction time in discrete response tasks.

The transfer functions relating to δ_w and Ψ_a are

$$\delta_w = K \int \Psi_a (t - \tau) \, dt, \text{ in the time } (t) \text{ domain, and}$$

$$\frac{\delta_q}{\Psi_a} = Ke - \tau j\omega, \text{ in the complex frequency } (j\omega) \text{ domain.}$$

In actual practice, the driver's output is not entirely dependent on the input, and so it was necessary to include a 'remnant' term in the final expression of the model. The contribution of the remnant is seen as driver-generated noise by the model's inventors, but its recognition by them should alert anyone to the possibility that human tracking behaviour is not exclusively determined by the perceptual input.

Traditionally, driver gain and transmission lag have been measured using a particular driving simulator test paradigm. The driver attempts to hold a steady course while his 'vehicle' is occasionally 'buffeted' by the application of a sum of sine wave inputs simulating the visual effect of a sudden gust of crosswind. The driver's compensatory steering-wheel movement is measured and later decomposed into components at each of the input frequencies. The corresponding output : input ratios are calculated in dB (log) units, as are the phase shifts from input to output signals. These variables are described as separate functions of log frequency in respective parts of a Bode plot.

If the driver has responded as a first-order system controller, the amplitude ratio is highly positive at the lowest input frequency and diminishes in linear manner over log frequency. The ratio is one (i.e., output = input) at some particular frequency (the crossover, ω_0) and becomes increasingly smaller at higher frequencies. the gain constant, K, is the curve's intercept constant in this representation. Changes of K between tests move the curve up or down, thereby changing ω_0 proportionately, but leave the slope unchanged.

Pure first-order control necessarily involves an integration phase lag of $90°$. At very low input frequencies this factor is practically all that determines the phase shift. The driver's transmission lag, however, adds progressively to the phase shift as frequency rises. The result on the Bode plot is an exponentially increasing phase shift as a function of log frequency. The transmission lag, τ, is the rate constant in this representation. Its minimum value is assumed to hold while the driver performs the task in an optimal condition. Factors that increase $\hat{\tau}$ would cause a more rapid increase in phase shift with increasing lag frequency. When this occurs the critical frequency where the output lags the input by $180°$ is lower than normal.

Tracking performance in any first-order control system which has an appreciable transmission lag must be a U-shaped function of gain. In other words, there is an optimal gain for the particular system. Lower gain produces a sluggish response which prolongs the error, and higher gain increases the likelihood of instability. The latter occurs as the combined result of high gain and long lag. If an output : input ratio exceeding unity can occur in conjunction with a phase shift of $180°$, then the system will become unstable when responding to the corresponding frequency input. This is because the output intended to reduce the input at the frequency will, by the time it is realized, add to the error rather than subtract from it.

The implications of the crossover model for interpreting sedative drug effects on a driver's tracking performance are straightforward. Such drugs are known to lengthen reaction time and, by analogy, should affect the driver's transmission lag in exactly the same way. This alone would be enough to create certain problems in vehicle handling. In the frequency domain, the phase shift between error input and response output would increase. Unless there is a compensatory drop in gain, their will be a greater likelihood of instability when the driver is suddenly forced to engage in evasive manoeuvres requiring high-frequency error correction. The time required to correct any error also increases exponentially with increasing transmission lag. Thus, the error amplitude would be larger over time during simple straight road tracking, leading to larger lateral position variability.

In psychophysiological terms, gain can be conceived as the factor governing the rate and amplitude of motor activation during a response. It would hardly be surprising if a sedative drug's effect was to reduce gain as well as increase transmission lag by diminishing activation in the systems that support both processes. If this occurs, the driver's response to error signals would not only be delayed but also less in amplitude. Corrections would be even slower, errors would persist longer, and lateral position variability would increase further. Although this might reduce the danger of instability, the driver would simply be unable to respond effectively to high-frequency error inputs which were formerly within the region of his compensatory response.

There was some evidence for reduced gain in a group of subjects treated daily with 15 mg diazepam for nine days and challenged on the last day with a dose of ethanol sufficient to raise maximum blood alcohol concentrations to about 0.10% (Moskowitz and Smiley, 1982). Additional groups of subjects were treated with 20 mg buspirone daily or with placebo. These latter groups were otherwise handled in the same way as the former. The subjects' dynamic open-loop responses to wind buffeting in a driving simulator test were determined to derive measures of the crossover frequency (ω_0) and the coherence (r) between the imposed heading angle error signal (input) and compensatory heading angle response (output) Some pertinent results are shown in Table 1.

Except after the alcohol challenge (ninth day post dose), mean ω_0 for the placebo group was stable around a value of 1.3 rad/s. The mean ω_0 for the

Table 1. Drivers' average dynamic responses in a simulator test (from Moskowitz and Smiley, 1982).

	Buspirone		Placebo		Diazepam	
	ω_0 (rad/sec)	r	ω_0 (rad/sec)	r	ω_0 (rad/sec)	r
1st day postdose	1.3	0.89	1.3	0.91	1.1	0.88
8th day predose	1.5	0.88	1.4	0.86	1.3	0.90
8th day postdose	1.3	0.89	1.3	0.90	1.0	0.83
9th day postdose	1.2	0.86	1.1	0.86	1.0	0.83

buspirone group was not significantly different. The mean ω_0 for the diazepam group, however, was significantly lower after both the first and eighth dose (15% and 23%). If the assumptions of the crossover model were met, this indicates proportional reductions in the group's gain. There may have been similar differences between the groups' average transmission lags, and this would presumably have been apparent from an analysis of input-output phase shifts. But if the authors did conduct such an analysis, they failed to report the results.

Coherence differences were generally nonsignificant, the only exception being that measured between the placebo and diazepam groups after the eight dose. This could have occurred if the contribution of the driver's remnant, or self-generated output variability, was greater in the latter group.

Before leaving the crossover model, it would be well to linger on the question of the remnant's importance. Although not clearly shown in the above results, a drug's effect could conceivably be to increase a driver's random steering-wheel output. This would produce a higher error amplitude within the closed-loop feedback system operating during continuous road tracking. The above-mentioned changes in the driver's gain and lag would render him less able to cope with the error of his own making. This insidious possibility suggests that it is not enough simply to consider the remnant as noise. It may in fact be the result of important processes, subject to the influence of drugs and other factors. The failure of the crossover model to examine this possibility is one of its chief weaknesses.

Variations of the Crossover Model

The original crossover model portrayed the drivers' tracking task as continuous. It may be that the motor output effecting steering-wheel control is continuous, or appears so from the close coupling between the driver and a steering system which under some circumstances generates its own torque. Yet experienced drivers certainly do not have the impression that they are continuously responding to an error signal in effecting their motor response. Discontinuities between episodes of closed-loop road tracking must occur as the driver attends to some other aspect of the driving task. Subsequent model builders have even suggested that there are discontinuities within closed-loop tracking itself.

Even within the limited human frequency bandwidth, the error signal must exceed a perceptual threshold before a response can be made. The operator may have to decide whether or not to react, and such discrete events are known to take time, during which already initiated movements may continue or be suppressed. For whatever reason, the operator may simply choose not to react to a well-perceived error signal until its amplitude exceeds a response criterion threshold. Finally, periods may occur in which the throughput of all information in the operator simply ceases, and the link between input and output is temporarily lost.

Recognition of these potential discontinuities has led theorists to propose revisions of the crossover model insofar as it pertains to driving. The first was by Carson and Weirwille (1978), who proposed that there is an interval of indifference around the amplitude of the error signal which must be exceeded within a certain fixed interval before a compensatory response is begun. The width of the band is determined by the perceptual threshold for detecting error changes, or by the response criterion, if these are not the same. The authors were able to estimate from empirical data the values of the physical factors of lateral position and heading angle changes which are associated with the width of the error signal's indifference interval, ± 0.15 m and $\pm 0.27°$ respectively.

Carson and Wierwille's model defines a continuously operating control system, but one with a nonlinear input-output relationship. Once an output has nulled a particular error input, the input is sustained until feedback indicates that the subsequent error amplitude has exceeded the limit of the indifference interval. The output is then once more modified accordingly.

If this model is essentially valid, any drug which raises thresholds that are relevant to perception of the error signal should impair tracking performance. Again it is hard to imagine such perceptual changes as correlates of mild sedation. Yet a sedative drug might very well raise the response criterion to achieve precisely the same effect.

Baxter and Harrison (1979) were more concerned with the ambiguity of the crossover model's remnant, believing that at least some of the seemingly random part of the output could be the result of an important process within the driver. They modelled this process in the mathematical form of a hysteresis loop which was then used as a multiplicative factor attached to the usual gain constant in the crossover model. Their hysteresis loop has its own periodic frequency and amplitude characteristics which modulate gain and thence the output, irrespective of the input. In the case of tracking an absolutely straight road, where the crossover model would predict no lateral position variance were it not for the remnant, the hysteresis model predicts periodic changes first in heading angle and second in lateral position. Taking vehicular dynamics into account, the latter model furthermore predicts a relationship between the periodic output due to hysteresis and speed, i.e., increasing frequency and diminishing amplitude with increasing speed. Both of these predictions were confirmed in experiments, though the overall difference between their model's predictions and those of the crossover model were only slightly in their favour.

At this point one should ask how any man-machine system can possibly benefit through the operation of an internally generated hysteresis loop. This could occur, however, if the driver's self-generated oscillatory output affects the vehicle-road system such that his perceptual system is sensitized to the detection or error signals related to movement of the visual scene. A modern theory of driver perception (Riemersma, 1982) holds that the error signals are (a) the rotation of the entire visual scene due to lateral vehicle movement, (b) the lateral translation of the same due to angular vehicle moment, and (c) lateral position deviation from the road boundaries. The former two signals are acted upon more or less continuously to permit smooth tracking, and the latter only at discrete points in time for realigning the vehicle's position for the resumption of continuous tracking.

If this theory is correct, then responding to the error signal largely depends upon the driver's acquisition of kinematic information arising from the vehicle-road interaction. It could even be said that the perception of motion is at all times necessary for efficient control. If the vehicle were to leave the road at a divergent heading angle too small to result in the crossing of a visual motion threshold, then the situation would go uncorrected until the driver's perception of a rather extreme lateral position elicited a discrete realignment response. Over time, the driver's road tracking performance would describe a sawtooth pattern of lateral movement. On the other hand, if tracking any straight tangent were accomplished with internally produced oscillation, the error signal would comprise a component related to the oscillation. The components would alternately cancel and sum. During summation, motion perception leading to a compensatory response would be enhanced. Moreover, the required direction for the response would often be the same as the next half cycle of the hysteresis output. The compensatory response would be smoother and more rapid as a consequence.

Hysteresis could cause a problem if its contribution to the output were to grow. This would defeat the apparent purpose of hysteresis by adding unduly to the error signal. Hysteresis frequency must also be closely coupled to the vehicle's speed. It should increase with speed with a corresponding drop in amplitude so that self-induced angular and lateral velocities will remain constant. This was actually confirmed by Baxter and Harrison (1979) for drivers operating normally on straight road tangents. But if it did not occur, low-frequency high-amplitude hysteresis, adding to a high-frequency high-amplitude disturbance, could conceivably produce an error situation beyond the driver's control.

A sedative drug might alter both the amplitude and frequency of hysteresis in a manner producing large oscillations inappropriate to the vehicle's speed. It may be simple to determine if this is the case, since according to Baxter and Harrison, the modal frequency of steering-wheel movements during straight road tracking is a valid index of the hysteresis frequency. Their model specifies an optimum frequency and its relationship to speed. If a driver's modal steering-wheel movement frequency fails to conform to that specified by the model after he receives a sedative drug, this would be evidence that inappropriate hysteresis is the factor responsible for his degraded tracking performance.

The number of possible explanations for the common effect of sedative drugs has grown with the introduction of the latest model (Blaauw, 1984). The Supervisory Driver Model describes two levels of information processing responsible for road tracking performance. The bottom—or control—level contains essentially the same stages of information processing as appear in continuous, closed-loop or servocontrol models. That is, the first stage is involved in perception of the error signal, and the final stage in the control of motor output. It is conceivable that Blaauw's system can operate in continuous closed-loop control, but it need not, owing to another function allocated to the perceptual stage and the role delegated to the top—or decision—level.

The perceptual process in Blaauw's model also extrapolates the error signal forward in time. Extrapolations occur successively at a high rate, varying one to the next in a stochastic manner. These are directed to a limited storage compartment on the decision level, where they are processed to yield the most probable extrapolation and a variance of extrapolations (uncertainty). Nothing further occurs on this level until the most probable extrapolation indicates the occurrence of an unacceptable error or the degree of uncertainty exceeds some threshold. At this point a decision process is activated which interrupts an ongoing control activity to force a discrete compensatory motor response. Blaauw leads one to infer that only the decision process is 'conscious' and pre-emptive of other information processing by the driver. Thus, for most of the driving task only a small part of the driver's total capacity is directly involved in vehicular guidance.

Blaauw conducted a series of simulator and actual driving tests to provide evidence in support of his model. He employed a visual occlusion technique which forced the drivers to go from closed-loop to open-loop control and measured the time before their increasing uncertainty caused them to remove the occlusion. He further varied vehicle speed and road curvature to show the predicted effects of these factors on the duration of voluntary visual occlusion.

The results showed that it is possible for drivers to achieve a reasonable degree of control precision while alternating between closed-loop and open-loop operation. Motor programmes which are in progress at the beginning of occlusion simply continue until the decision to remove it. When this occurs the drivers make a discrete response, if required, but otherwise resume closed-loop operation without noticeably altering their output. Blaauw suggests that it might be quite normal for experienced drivers to alternate between closed-loop operation in conjunction with decision and open-loop operation between decisions. This model explains very nicely why the task of road tracking seems so simple for experienced drivers. Most of the time is spent with the system operating open-loop through the execution of well-practised motor programmes. Higher, capacity-consuming processes are only involved intermittently and remain mainly free for monitoring functions or for engaging in activities irrelevant to driving. Without recourse to the artificial visual occlusion technique, however, it is seemingly impossible to determine when decisions are made. Their rate during experimental trials may correspond to their normal rate in actual driving, but there is no assurance of this.

In any case, Blaauw demonstrated that continuous closed-loop control of lateral position is not necessary for efficient road tracking. His empirical studies, as much of his theory, call all of the older models into question. If a driver cannot be modelled in terms of a continuous servocontrol system, then the alternative is to postulate various cognitive mechanisms such as decision making. These may operate according to principles which may eventually be defined as rigorously as the relatively simple servocontrol systems, but for the present one can only speculate about the means for measuring their functions.

It may be that sedative drug effects only occur within higher control mechanisms. One may assume that intermittent control asserted by some decision process occurs at intervals that describe something like a Poisson distribution over time. Such a distribution would have a strict limit at the lower end as determined by the minimal decision-making interval. There is no limit at the other end, however, short of the interval that, depending on vehicle speed and road geometry, just permits the driver to correct his error before the vehicle leaves the road. Factors which separately retard the decision-making process should increase the mean interval between successive compensatory responses, while their variance increases in proportion to the square of the mean. Thus, the vehicle's path over time should not show periodic lateral motion but instead a mixture of short, long, and occasionally very long intervals when error accumulates, each followed by corrective manoeuvres which are short relative to the periods of increasing error that precede them. The increase in lateral position variance would be proportional to the increase in decision interval variance. It should be an easy matter to determine whether changes in lateral position variability under the influence of sedative drugs are mainly periodic or nonperiodic by nature. In the former case, the results would support the validity of the earlier models, whereas the latter results would favour Blaauw's model.

In conclusion, any of the described driver performance models can be used to explain the common effect of sedative drugs on lateral position variability during road tracking in the standard test. Each model makes different assumptions about the processes involved, and it is unlikely that they can all be correct. Nonetheless, there seem to be both experimental and analytical means of selecting the model that most plausibly explains the effect of sedative drugs on road tracking ability.

A Possible Research Programme

From the preceding discussion we have identified the following variables which might be influenced by drugs, either separately or in some combination:

1. Gain
2. Transmission lag
3. Perceptual threshold
4. Response criterion
5. Driver-generated hysteresis
6. Decision-making frequency

A programme of research to investigate possible drug effects on each of these variables could be systematically organized in the following manner. The involvement of gain and transmission lag should first be ascertained using the classic 'wind gust' test paradigm described above. The subject's open-loop compensatory responses to imposed perturbations can be analysed in the usual manner to reveal changes in their gains and lags under the influence of drugs. Yet this approach also has its limitations: the subject's output is so closely linked to the imposed input that almost no spontaneously generated output, implying the operation of another variable, can ever be observed. Moreover, the necessity of repeatedly perturbing the system to generate enough data for obtaining average variable estimates in reasonably short tests practically guarantees that the subject will be performing close to the limits of his capacity for whatever physiological state he is in at the time. None of the effects of time on task or dual task interference, which almost certainly occur in this experimental situation, is considered. Nonetheless, such a gross effect as increased transmission lag, analogous to slower reaction time, can be observed. In the absence of such changes, one can safely discount this possibility while seeking other sources of impaired performance.

Perceptual impairments can be investigated once it becomes possible to specify the perceptual error signal which normally constitutes the driver's control input. A plausible approach would be to employ a computer model for constructing the usual imagery of straight and curve driving for presentation to subjects in a driving simulator. The subjects would not interact with the system but would instead respond whenever they perceive that the vehicle has embarked on a course which, if left uncorrected, would eventually lead to the car's leaving the road. The average amplitude of the error signal at these times could then be taken as indicating a perceptual threshold. Repeated applications of this procedure after the subjects have been treated with placebo and different doses of a drug should show whether the drug can be expected to alter driver perception.

A variation of this approach could be applied to measure the drug's effects on the response criterion. In this case the subjects would follow the same scenario while themselves in closed-loop control of the system and its displayed imagery. The average amplitude of the error signal at times when the subject effects steering-wheel reversals could be taken as a measure of his response criterion. Because perceptual threshold and response criterion would presumably be measured under comparable treatment conditions in the same study, its results should separate drug effects on the two parameters.

It may only be possible to measure a change in the hysteresis process during actual car driving or a near perfect simulation thereof. This is because such a process would be heavily dependent upon vehicular dynamics as these affect the driver's visual and perhaps proprioceptive inputs in continuous closed-loop operation. Yet even if one were to observe changes in the driver's oscillatory output under the influence of drugs, one would still be unable to ascribe these to hysteresis changes. They could just as easily result from alterations in gain and lag as predicted by the classic crossover model. To discount the latter possibilities, it would be necessary to perturb the motion of the vehicle occasionally and determine that gain and lag remain unchanged while oscillatory output is elevated between the perturbations.

It is difficult to conceive of tests which unambiguously measure the decision process in drivers operating in traffic on normal roads. A drug-induced slowing of the decision process could lead to greater tracking error, since the system must operate open-loop for longer periods. On the other hand, more frequent decisions followed by closed-loop compensatory responses could occur if the driver became aware of a drug's influence. Thus, the decision rate could be affected in either direction in the same or different individuals. To determine the true state of affairs it would be necessary to somehow measure the occurrence of decisions, whether or not they are followed by responses, and to ask the driver for his impression of how much effort was involved in driving.

Much of the process of perceiving tracking error seems to depend upon movement of the entire visual field. One part of error perception, however, may depend upon the occasional visual fixations that allow the driver to judge the distance of his vehicle from road boundaries and to reset his course if necessary. The measurement of eye fixation may, in this case, provide indices of the decision frequency and the durations of individual decisions. Of course, only some of these fixations will result in a decision leading to a movement of the steering-wheel. But even if a fraction of fixations at a certain place in the visual field are followed shortly by a characteristic response, it may be assumed that the others occurring at the same place were also followed by a decision (not to respond in the latter case). Careful studies of eye movements in relation to steering-wheel movements will be necessary to establish the relationship between fixations at a particular place and the occurrence of clearly associated responses. If this approach should fail, the only apparent procedure for inferring the operation of a decision process would be through an analysis of the temporal pattern of compensatory reactions, as suggested earlier.

Conclusions

The fact that many sedative drugs cause drivers to allow an increase in the SD lateral position of their vehicle during uninterrupted high-speed travel is an established phenomenon in search of an explanation. Current models of driver performance can all be used to provide plausible explanations, though they differ from model to model and cannot all be valid. Yet each model can be used to predict an unique set of phenomena associated with elevated SD lateral position. There seems to be a need for a systematic comparison of the models' predictive validity to account fully for the behavioural effects. The required research programme would probably involve a number of experimental and analytical approaches using various behavioural and physiological test procedures. Laboratory, driving simulator, and actual driving performance tests would all be required for a comprehensive evaluation of competing models. This research would be both costly and time-consuming, yet its success would fully justify the effort. The model which best explains the phenomenon may be the best representation of road tracking behaviour under any circumstance. Moreover, the variables of such a model, once identified as psychophysiological processes residing in biological mechanisms, would allow one to better define the nature of the effects of sedative drugs. The conclusion of a successful programme would therefore simultaneously advance concepts in two areas: human performance modelling and psychopharmacology.

References

Baxter J and Harrison JY (1979) A non-linear model describing driver behaviour on straight roads. *Hum. Factors* **21**, 87–97.

Blaauw GJ (1984) *Car Driving as a Supervisory Control Task* (doctoral dissertation). Soesterberg, The Netherlands: Institute for perception TNO.

Carson JM and Weirwille WW (1978) Development of a strategy model of the driver in lane keeping. *Vehicle System Dynamics* **7**, 223–53.

McRuer DT and Weir DH (1969) Theory of manual vehicular control. *Ergonomics* **12**, 599–633.

McRuer DT, Weir DH, Jex HR, Magdaleno RE and Allen RW (1975) Measurement of driver-vehicle multiloop response properties with a single disturbance input. *IEEE Trans. Systems, Man and Cybernetics*, S.M.C. **5**, 490–7.

Moskowitz H and Smiley A (1982) Effects of chronically administered buspirone and diazepam on driving-related skills performance. *J. Clin. Psychiatry* **43**, 44–55.

O'Hanlon JF (1986) Application of actual driving tests in drug registration procedures. In: O'Hanlon JF and de Gier JJ (eds.) *Drugs and Driving Performance*. London: Taylor and Francis.

Riemersma JBJ (1982) Perceptual cues in vehicle guidance on a straight road. *Proceedings, 2nd European annual manual*. Conference on Human Decision Making and Control FGAN/FAT, Bonn, FRG.

Weir DH and McRuer DT (1968) A theory for driver steering control of motor vehicles. *Highway Research Board* **247**, 7–39.

Wier DH and McRuer DT (1973) Measurement and interpretation of driver/vehicle system dynamic response. *Hum. Factors* **15**, 367–78.

Index